Religious Literacy in Hospice Care

This is the first book to explore how religion, belief and spirituality are negotiated in hospice care. Specifically, it considers the significant place that spiritual care has in hospice care and claims that the changing role of religion and belief in society highlights the need to re-examine how such identities are integrated in professional practice.

Using religious literacy as a framework, the author explores how healthcare professionals in hospice care respond to religion, belief and spiritual identities of service users. Part 1 provides a comprehensive account of the content and history of the place of religion, belief and spirituality in hospice care. Part 2 examines how these topics are negotiated in hospice care by looking at three key areas: environment, professional practice and organisation. Part 3 proposes a religious literacy model applicable to hospice care and explores implications for practice and policy. Lastly, the author identifies future trends in research, policy and practice.

Drawing on a range of theories and concepts, and proposing a working model that can impact the training of future and current professionals, *Religious Literary in Hospice Care* should be considered essential reading for students, researchers and practitioners.

Panagiotis Pentaris is a Senior Lecturer for the Department of Psychology, Social Work and Counselling at the University of Greenwich. He is also a Postdoc Research Fellow for the Faiths & Civil Society Unit at Goldsmiths, University of London. Panagiotis is a thanatologist, as well as a qualified social worker with specialty in hospice social work and clinical social work in end of life care. His research stretches from death policies to professional practice, and he has researched extensively about religion, belief and spirituality in end of life care.

Religious Literacy
in Hospice Care
Challenges and Controversies

Panagiotis Pentaris

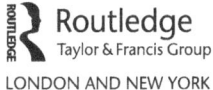

Routledge
Taylor & Francis Group

LONDON AND NEW YORK

First published 2019
by Routledge
2 Park Square, Milton Park, Abingdon, Oxon OX14 4RN

and by Routledge
52 Vanderbilt Avenue, New York, NY 10017

First issued in paperback 2020

*Routledge is an imprint of the Taylor & Francis Group,
an informa business*

British Library Cataloguing-in-Publication Data
A catalogue record for this book is available from the British Library.

Library of Congress Cataloging-in-Publication Data
Names: Pentaris, Panagiotis, author.
Title: Religious literacy in hospice care : challenges and controversies /
Panagiotis Pentaris.
Other titles: Religious literacy in end of life care
Description: Abingdon, Oxon ; New York, NY : Routledge, 2018. |
Revision of author's thesis (doctoral)—Goldsmiths University of
London, 2015 titled
Religious literacy in end of life care : challenges and controversies. |
Includes bibliographical references and index.
Identifiers: LCCN 2018022716 | ISBN 9781138477957 (hardback) |
ISBN 9781351103732 (ebook)
Subjects: LCSH: Hospice care—Religious aspects. | Terminal
care—Religious aspects.

ISBN 13: 978-0-36-758514-3 (pbk)
ISBN 13: 978-1-138-47795-7 (hbk)

Typeset in Times NR MT Pro
by Cenveo® Publisher Services

In memory of Stratos Mpouzounierakis

Contents

List of figures

List of tables

Acknowledgements

This book would not have been possible without the support and guidance that I received from many people, starting with those who supported me during my PhD, which is the basis of this monograph.

First and foremost, I thank my PhD advisor, Professor Adam Dinham. Professor Dinham not only supported and guided me to complete my thesis and, later, conceptualise it in the form of a book, but also he has been a mentor to me, encouraging my ambitions and aspirations, and allowing me to become the researcher and academic I have become. I am also thankful for the exceptional example he has been to me. His advice on both research as well as my career has been priceless.

I gratefully acknowledge the funding received during my PhD studies from the State Scholarship Institute in Greece (Ίδρυμα Κρατικών Υποτροφιών Ελλάδος – IKY). Thanks to the staff of the Institute for all their support during this PhD fellowship. Without this funding, the project would not have been completed and this book would not have come to life. I also greatly appreciate the support received from hospice trusts in London during the fieldwork. The excellent collaboration during data collection truly supported the completion of the project, which then informed this book. I am thankful to all hospice professionals who kindly engaged with my research and supported my understanding of how religion and belief are negotiated in hospice care.

I also give a heartfelt thank you to my sister, Rena Gatzounis, for always believing in me and encouraging me to pursue my dreams and fulfil my aspirations. Rena, you have always been a role model to me and have always taught me that 'there is a way'. Special thanks and my love to my partner, Jeffrey Baker, who gave me the space to work on this book and read drafts, and our son, Jack Pentaris Baker, for supporting me during this challenging period of authoring my first book. Jack kindly endured my long weekends of writing. He supported me in his own special and priceless way. I am forever grateful to him and the lessons he teaches me every day.

List of abbreviations

BR	Beveridge Report
BSA	British Social Attitudes
CLF	Chaplaincy Leadership Forum
DDB	Death, Dying and Bereavement
DH	Department of Health
DHSC	Department of Health and Social Care
EDS	Equality Delivery System
EHRC	Equality and Human Rights Commission
EOAP	Equality Objectives Action Plan
EOL	End of Life
HCPC	Health and Care Professions Council
HELP	Hospitalised Elderly Longitudinal Project
LCP	Liverpool Care Pathway
NEoLCIN	National End of Life Care Intelligence Network
NHS	National Health System
NPSRC	Network for Pastoral, Spiritual and Religious Care in Health
PHE	Public Health England
PPCP	Preferred Place of Care Plan
RLIIC	Religious Literacy for Hospice Care
SFPC	Solution-Focused Pastoral Counselling
SUPPORT	Study to Understand Prognoses and Preferences for Outcomes and Risks of Treatment
WHO	World Health Organization

Introduction

For decades, scholars have explored how we die and grieve; what makes our grief more, or less, tense and how we tend to respond to the losses we experience periodically in life; and how we can best care for those who are dying or grieving. Included in these explorations is the debate about the place of religion and belief in the care of the dying and bereaved. For centuries, religion has been a critical informant of both the nature and outcomes of death. Religion played a big part in the process of understanding death and dying, and appreciating the impact on the living and life. With that, religion has been an important part of people's support system; their faith often helps them make sense of their world and their experiences, inclusive of life itself. Equally, religion has been a source of knowledge when science and technology fail to explain several aspects of this human experience. Religious institutions and religious leaders, as well as believers, have always cared for the dying and those diagnosed with a life-threatening or life-limiting condition in societies across the world – and still do.

If religion plays such a big part in people's lives, how do we take it into account in contemporary practises when caring for the dying and bereaved? Similarly, how does contemporary hospice practise recognise the modern and post-modern perceptions about religion, informed by the different ways in which people believe nowadays, or identify with nonreligion and nonbelief? Cicely Saunders, a pioneer of hospice care, set strict parameters about the dimensions of hospice care, one of which emphasised the need for spiritual care and proper accommodation of service users' needs associated with their beliefs, religious or not. *Religious Literacy in Hospice Care: Challenges and Controversies* starts from this emphasis but moves beyond the hospice movement's intentions and examines the tensions between current religious changes and hospice practises.

This is a difficult task to undertake, though. To begin with, current hospice practises cannot be understood without a firm appreciation of their history and development. It is, in other words, the developing history of how religion and belief played out in the care of the dying that unravels from this argument. Such progression faces numerous challenges, however – the nature and quality of life, the nature of death, the meaning of death, and the meaning-making process through religious and nonreligious beliefs, to name a few.

Conversations about death

In accordance with Martin Heidegger's thoughts, one's conception of life in the knowledge of death is a liberating one (Heidegger, 1962; also see Edwards, Freeman and Sugden, 1979). However, death has for a long time been an unwelcome subject at the dinner table, and this is the outcome of the limited opportunities we are offered to become familiar with death nowadays. Until the mid-20th century, by and large, people would die at home. This tendency has since changed in the western world. The death site is no longer in the comfort of one's home; it is placed in hospitals, hospices or elderly homes (more than 80% of deaths in 2013[1]). Our detachment from death has led to a lack of conversation about death, as this is often treated as a medicalised subject – medicalised because the focus has shifted towards the prolongation or preservation of life but not always to increase the quality of life.

Philippe Aries (1974) accentuates the philosophical belief that death, towards the second half of the 20th century, is primarily a reminder of our mortal selves and 'foreign to our existential pessimism' (p. 44). This perception and ambivalence about conversing on this subject have changed throughout modern history. About 20 years earlier, in 1955, Geoffrey Gorer challenged death talk in public, though without significant impact until the 1980s. With his 'The Pornography of Death', Gorer (1955) describes societies being ambivalent to accommodate death talk – death being an issue that has had an immense impact on society after World Wars I and II. The same ambivalence is evident for half a century, as death in the 21st century is a subject for study, but not necessarily a part of life that people talk about comfortably. To fully appreciate the course that death talk has taken in time, and the ways in which it has influenced end of life (EOL) care, inclusive of hospice care, it is essential to familiarise oneself with death studies and hospice care, and their historical and developmental aspects.

Recalling Weber's identification (Weber, 1978) of the scientific era, technology and science have dominated in modern societies concerning death and dying; prolongation of life became more important than acceptance of its end. Death began to be considered a failure, a weakness of the body and a state of imperfection that is undoubtedly related to ageing (Morin, 1951; Feifel, 1959; Elias, 1985; Kastenbaum, 2000). Biomedical and clinical approaches to death have been gaining ground all through the 21st century (Kastenbaum, 2007; Emanuel and Librach, 2011; Ghesquiere et al, 2015), with grief models highlighting the dominance of clinical classification of the meaning-making process and experiences of dying and grieving (Wright and Hogan, 2008). Concurrently, the psychosocial study of experiences related to dying and grieving was ignored (Fonseca and Testoni, 2011–2012).

There are at least two repositories of conversation about death and dying that are happening separately but simultaneously. Existential philosophers have been developing discussions about death and dying prompted by the wars in the first half of the 20th century. Important works of these philosophically driven discussions about death include the following: American psychologist Herman Feifel (1959), one of the pioneers in death talk in the mid-20th century, and well-known Austrian neurologist Sigmund Freud, who became the founder of psychoanalysis. Freud (1915) was concerned with two difficulties which wars placed upon humanity. The first was disillusionment, arguing that we ought to set aside our sentimentality and accept that wars will never cease to occur. The second was the changing attitudes towards death that were forced upon people due to the multitude of losses associated with war, as well as the frequency with which losses occur. Freud's talk about losses, death and war signified the extension of this dialogue beyond the period of war. After both World Wars ended, Feifel (1959) reflected on the aftermath of the losses the first half of the 20th century brought and prompted the dialogue about death further, examining the meanings of death beyond the wars. Freud and Feifel are but two examples of those who engaged in such conversations during that period.

A second discourse is taking place in theology and religious studies about death and life. Pattison (2013) offers a critical theological reflection of death, the meaning of death in modern societies and the afterlife. Pattison (2013) bases his analysis on Heidegger's philosophy about death. Such reflections add to the argument about how religion and belief are associated with death as an experience and as a concept for discussion.

The review of the religious discourse about death shows us that concerns about the meaning of death in life, post-death experiences and resurrection have always been present in the discussions (Van Baaren, 1967). Westphal (1984) identifies two main problems with human life which link to religious discourse too: guilt and death. In his theological analysis, he explains what it means to be religious whilst attempting to resolve guilt and death. He offers an analytical account of the intersection of religious belief and the experience of dying and being lost. It is often the relationship between death and religion that intensifies guilt, which later impacts one's sense of worthiness to believe and thereafter die a 'good death', whatever the latter means.

The discourse about death in theology, parallel to Christian values and the Church, has been influential in Cicely Saunders' work when conceptualising and introducing hospice care (Saunders, 2005). Hospice care became a movement that received immeasurable influence by theological understandings of spiritual care, drawing from the values of social solidarity and humane approaches to promoting wellbeing and the quality of one's life. However, the care of the dying remained an attempt to cure the patient instead. It is a struggle, even today, to accept someone's *dying status* and allow them the comfort to die peacefully, as opposed to subjecting them to a medical profession's inherent need to preserve and save life.

The conversation has separated, and scientific observations and explanations about death dominate whilst ontological interpretations are avoided and pushed into the existential realm of human life (for a thanatological analysis of this, see Becker, 1971). This split in the conversation also splits the experience of the patients in hospice care, however. The first signs of awareness of this problem are the medical model, which gives way, first, to social work theories in the 1980s.

In his work, Carl Rogers (1979) expanded on a person-centred approach – namely, the client-centred theory. Since its beginning, the social work profession has followed the principles of a person-centred approach, based on the observations of social work practitioners that an individual's correspondence to life is unique and individualistic. Nelsen (1980), in *Communication Theory and Social Work Practice*, underscores the fragility of human beings in a complex environment, and the extensive need for a more humane, holistic and compassionate approach towards vulnerable situations. According to Donnison (1980), social work became a beacon of principles towards wellbeing of individuals. Herbert (1980) suggests "informed eclecticism" for social workers, alongside the wide range of professions that aim at social and health wellbeing of individuals and communities.

Subsequently, professional literature on death studies started reflecting on general policies, such as service user empowerment and children's rights. This consideration translates into death policies in the 21st century that are challenging the medical model and clinical approaches in hospice and palliative care. The End of Life Care Strategy 2008 in the UK comes first to identify explicitly the needs of patients towards the end of their lives. The strategy also signifies the importance of a holistic approach to care and enhancement of the experience of patients, whilst involving compassionate perspectives in care. In the prime of this discourse, death policies are now informed by conversations about spirituality, compassion and wellbeing, all introduced as remedies to psychosocial, emotional and religious needs of patients. NHS Improving Quality of Care, in 2012, assesses and improves the quality of healthcare altogether, including hospice and palliative care. This initiative promotes the principles of wellbeing and spiritual understanding of patients by hospice professionals.

Spiritual care

Spiritual care is recognised largely in the healthcare system (Department of Health, 2009) whilst its presence has been challenged (Walter, 2002). In the past 20 years, professional literature has focussed on the spiritual needs of patients (Stanworth, 2004; McSherry and Ross, 2010) and wellbeing as a vital dimension of the quality of care (Jewell, 2004). This recognition is magnified in EOL care (Kuebler, Davis and Moore, 2005) and for various reasons. First and foremost, spirituality has been recognised as a patient need (Bulkley et al, 2013; Henoch et al, 2013). With equal importance, the conclusion has been reached that spirituality affects healthcare decision-making (Lucchetti, Bassi and Lucchetti, 2013; Gijsberts et al, 2013), whilst it influences healthcare outcomes, including quality of life (Exline et al, 2013; Cook and Silverman, 2013; Hess, 2013; Nelson-Becker, 2013; Healy, 2013).

The recognition of the importance of religion, belief and spirituality as core dimensions of hospice and palliative care can be found on various levels, one being policy-making. General policies and death policies in the UK have recently started recognising religion and belief as new strands for integration in health and social care (e.g., Public Health England, 2016). The Equality Act 2010 identifies religion and belief as one of the nine protective characteristics. This has a substantial effect on death policies as well (e.g., 'End of Life Care Strategy'; 'Improving Care'; 'Compassion in Practice'). The Act introduces religion and belief in the conversation, but the levels of knowledge and understanding to do so are questionable.

According to Dinham (2015), professionals and policy-makers struggle to have that conversation because of lack of religious literacy. There is an ill understanding of religion and belief which undermines the principles of holistic care and wellbeing in healthcare as a whole (also see Dinham and Francis, 2015), and in hospice care in particular (Pentaris, 2013). Religious literacy is neither an alternative nor a substitute for any of the concepts of 'religion', 'spirituality', 'nonreligion', 'belief', 'nonbelief' or 'faith'. Religious literacy is a contested notion that can only be understood within context. It refers to better skills and abilities to engage with religion and belief (Dinham and Francis, 2015). This argument, highlighted in Chapter 2 of this book, needs to be complemented by the history of religious change in the UK. For starters, Bryan Wilson (1966) suggested that religion lost its social significance as societies modernised. This started what is known as the secularisation thesis. Beginning in the mid-20th century, secularisation theories took hold, and secularism and the argument that religion and belief have been absent from the public sphere informed policy and practise. Nonetheless, as suggested by many, including Berger (1999), Dinham (2012) and Davie (2007), religion has maintained its social significance, both on individual and societal levels, regardless of the suggestions about the opposite. Exploring these dialogues and shifting public attitudes towards religion is a necessary task towards understanding that there is lack of religious literacy, a need for adequate health and death policies, and implementation of practises that meet individual needs on a holistic level.

At a time when religion and belief, after having experienced a prolonged period of public repudiation, are resurfacing in the public sphere, the study informing this book focusses on the influences that the secular characteristics of today's society have had on the healthcare service delivery system and, more specifically, on hospice care. It explores religious literacy in hospice care and in hospice professionals in Britain. The hypothesis that hospice professionals in Britain tend to be or are illiterate concerning religious matters emerges in the context of religion in relation to the state, in post-war

Britain (Wilson, 1976), the trend of privatisation of religious affairs over the same period, the relationship between the state and the Church (Davie, 1994, 2013), as well as the emergence of social welfare and the state as the commissioner of welfare services (Dinham, 2015).

Introducing this book

This book offers a rounded and comprehensive view of how religion, belief and spirituality (including nonreligion and nonbelief) are associated aspects of hospice care. The book decompartmentalises hospice care in three areas – space, professionals, and organisation; it examines how religion, belief and spirituality are present in or absent from these areas; and then it combines that knowledge to offer a more rounded view on the subject.

Intersecting thanatological and religious studies is an ambiguous task. In the past, many scholars examined aspects of death and dying via a religious and/or spiritual lens. Others explored religious belief from a death studies perspective. Fonseca and Testoni (2011–2012) have recently examined the literature about the emergence of thanatology in death education, alluding to the need for death education in practise as well. In their exploration, they opined that religion plays a vital part in how we experience death and grief, and stretched the importance to examine that intersection further.

Walter (1994) also attempted to touch on the intersection of the two fields aforementioned. His work examined the re-visitation and public re-conceptualisation of death via a Christian-centred lens and using a sociological exploration; though with no links to the sociology of religion, the subfield of sociology that examines the place of religion in societies. Davies (2013) is another example of a scholar whose work indeed intersects religion and death, but not methodologically or epistemologically. Davies' (2013) work is concerned with rituals and the anthropological enquiry of how death and bereavement are experienced through rituals as public expressions of feelings and emotions associated with the former. Grimes et al (2011) offer a similar account of rituals situated in the process of caring for the dead body, often in, or in the form of, funerary films.

Doka et al (2016) reviewed literature in thanatology since 1991 and reported on the trends of and epistemological evolvement in the field. Their review shows that interdisciplinary discourses in thanatology, or otherwise death studies, are on the rise. Equally, cross-national and international collaborations are increasing rapidly. Both these findings ascertain that scholars have not always had methodological and epistemological exchanges, which may have limited our understanding of various social phenomena. This book's argument is the product of the intersection of thanatological and religious studies; it examines how religion, belief and spirituality are integrated aspects of hospice care and EOL care altogether. To do so, it employs theoretical frames from the sociology of religion as well as other fields, like social work and anthropology of religion, and epistemologies from the field of sociology and anthropology. The use of theories from the sociology of religion, an area which has recently emerged and evolved (Davie, 2013), makes this volume unique and far from what previous scholars have accomplished.

Following a grant from the European Return Fund in 2012 and a scholarship from the Institute of Greek Scholarships in 2013, I started out to explore how we care for the dying and bereaved for whom religion, belief, spirituality or their identity of nonbelief are important. My interest was informed by my training in social work, medical psychology and thanatology. Equally, I was intrigued by the topic due to my experience in EOL care. Starting in 2012, I networked with many professionals and agencies that offer EOL care to in-patients, out-patients as well as in the community. Between 2013 and 2015, I collected data that answered my research questions, yet led me to leave the project with many more, as research does. Specifically, I visited more than 25 hospices in the Greater London Area of England, and some in the south of England. Also, I spent over 12 months and more than 25 hours per week in the role of an observer in two hospices in the Greater London Area. Further to my observations and informal interviews with various professionals in various hospices, I had the chance to carry out more than 40 in-depth interviews with hospice professionals as well as focus groups which brought professionals from different hospices together to share ideas and have debates.

This book is the most cohesive product from the project mentioned above. The research that I carried out provided me with the knowledge to write this book and present a clear image of how religion, belief and spirituality are integrated aspects of care in hospices. It also offered evidence that supported the development of a religious literacy model for hospice care (RLHC).

Terms and concepts

Undeniably, the literature on spiritual care, religion, belief and nonreligion has, by and large, occupied itself with definitional and conceptual enquiries. Scholars from across the world and various disciplines, and for decades, have engaged in exhaustive dialogue about the definitions and characteristics of each of the following terms: religion, nonreligion, spirituality, belief and nonbelief. The aim of this section is not to offer a thorough account of the various definitions of these terms, but to set clear how this book uses these terms and for what purpose.

This book accepts the unique context and content of each of the terms mentioned earlier, but also those that have not been mentioned, like faith. The book explores these terms based on the way they are conceptualised in the context in which they are explored, and calls for attention to universalism and more international perspectives about religion and belief altogether. In other words, this book does not aim at defining any of these terms but accepts that faith and belief are individual- and organisation-specific concepts, which can only be understood in the context in which they materialise. That said, religious literacy is also explored with care, due to its fluid character.

Last, for the purposes of this book, I refer to the terms religion, belief and spirituality to discuss all the various ways in which people identify (e.g., faith, nonreligious, etc.). Occasionally, I make further references to nonreligion and nonbelief, when necessary, to emphasise the arguments made.

Overview of the chapters

The structure of this book includes eight chapters divided into three parts. The first part contextualises the development of the argument of this book. The second part directly reports on findings from this study and presents a thorough analysis of them. The final part offers an analytical presentation of the model of RLHC.

Chapter 1 discusses the development of the hospice movement, the establishment of hospice care and the role of religion, belief and spirituality in modern hospice care. This chapter is the first of two which formulate the argument of this book. Readers will gain a complete and elaborate understanding of how religion and belief are in the grassroots of the hospice philosophy by exploring religious motivation in the care of people who are near the end of their lives. The chapter begins with an exploration of the progression of the hospice movement's development. It draws on Cicely Saunders' work and comments on how her Christian beliefs heavily influenced her motivation and decisions when promoting the whole care of a person towards the end of life. The chapter focuses on the concept of 'total pain' and identifies spirituality as one of its dimensions, and examines the links with interdisciplinary teams. From there, the chapter emphasises the place of religion, belief and spirituality in hospice care and modern practises.

Chapter 2 sketches how the role of religion has changed over time, focussing on the religious diversification of the British population and its impact on public life. It also draws on theoretical perspectives of religion and examines how these frame the book's arguments.

Specifically, the chapter begins with a discussion about religious plurality and religious diversification to emphasise the need for further and more elaborate approaches in practise and policy. It focusses on the UK but also uses examples from the US and Australia to stress the impact of religious plurality and diversification internationally. The text complements this discussion with references to the phenomenon of secularity and examines secularisation theories and how they impact on the contemporary understandings of religion and belief. Next, the chapter provides an exhaustive account of religious literacy; it examines the various descriptors of the concept and identifies its benefits and limitations. Last, the chapter negotiates how the frame of religious literacy has been used to make sense of this book's arguments.

Chapter 3 outlines the policy context in hospice care, focussing on religion, belief and spirituality. It analyses the key policy documents and how religion, belief and spirituality are placed in them. This is important to gain further insight on the guidelines that directly inform professional practise.

In more detail, the chapter begins with an exploration of policies pertinent to hospice care. This exploration gives evidence of how religion, belief and spirituality are negotiated aspects of care, as well as people's identities. The chapter provides a firm analysis of such documents (i.e., policies) and highlights the contested use of the terms religion, belief and spirituality in policy and how that shapes practise. The overall aim of the chapter is to set the policy context of how religion, belief and spirituality are integrated into the care of people near the end of their lives, or with conditions often threatening to their lives. This information better prepares readers to contrast the arguments of the second part of the book against the current policy framework as it shapes practise and provides a platform for drawing conclusions and highlighting future trends in the concluding section.

Chapters 4 through 7 provide a structured and comprehensive analysis of how religion, belief and spirituality are present in or absent from hospice care. These chapters present extracts from interviews, case studies and vignettes (all names are pseudonyms, for confidentiality purposes). Chapter 4 focuses on the presence and/or absence of religion, belief and spirituality in hospice care settings. The chapter provides case studies which illustrate how material objects are either present or not in a hospice's various spaces, such as units, wards and prayer rooms. The aim of this chapter is to illustrate how hospices accommodate religion, belief and spirituality by looking at religious material objects in the space of hospice care, as well as how professionals in hospice care use religious jewellery when in practise. Furthermore, this chapter examines this materiality using case studies that provide readers with helpful examples to further their learning and understanding. The chapter also shows how prayer rooms have been transformed, arguing that their purpose is changing and service users may retreat to other places for spiritual comfort. Specifically, Chapter 4 explores how prayer rooms have been used, by whom and who is using them today and why, and it uses vignettes to depict where service users have found comfort instead.

Chapter 5 examines definitional issues between religion and spirituality, as professional practitioners express them. It further explores similarities and differences between definitions and descriptions of the two, taking into account general definitions of religion and belief as found in the sociology of religion. In addition, the chapter focuses on discussing hospice professionals' views about the following: first, how religion, belief and spirituality are linked with the experiences of dying and grieving; and second, how far these identities are important to service users' lives. More specifically, the chapter examines how hospice professionals appreciate the significance that service users may place in their religion, belief or spiritual identity in relation to their experiences of dying and grieving. This information provides an initial account of what may be expected in practise and highlights further education needs or challenges, which are stressed in 'Conclusions'.

Chapter 6 describes hospice professionals' knowledge, understanding, skills and abilities to respond to religion, belief and spiritual-related needs of the dying and/or bereaved. The chapter examines the interplay between professionals' willingness to engage with care on this level and the ability to do so. In detail, it examines the depth and breadth of knowledge about religion, belief and spirituality that hospice professionals' views indicate. Drawing on literature and my research, this chapter explores two main areas. First, it studies the professionals' views about knowledge exchange in hospice care, which increases skills and abilities in practise. Second, it examines professional limitations and lack of understanding of religion and belief when providing care to people for whom religion, belief and spirituality are important. In summary, the chapter discusses practically how hospice professionals respond to service user needs related to religion, belief and spirituality.

Chapter 7 discusses how religion, belief and spirituality are integrated aspects of hospice care. It draws on my research in the field and highlights current practises and approaches towards religion, belief and spirituality. First, the chapter examines how death and health policies are inherently linked with what professionals do in the field and, complemented by the discussion in Chapter 3, this account stresses the imbalance between the loose use of terms and concepts in policy documents and how they materialise in practise. Next, the chapter explores assessment and religious networks to be essential ways in which professionals provide care pertaining to religion, belief and spiritual needs. Equally, the emphasis on neutrality in hospices is discussed to promote an inclusive environment for practise, as the chapter discusses. Furthermore, the chapter emphasises the binary between professionals' coping strategies and practise models to stress the complexity of achieving full and efficient integration of religion and belief in hospice care.

Chapter 8 does two things. First, it re-joins the concepts discussed in Chapters 4, 5, 6 and 7 in a concluding discussion about religious literacy in hospice care. Second, it introduces the model of religious literacy for hospice care. Each stage and level of the model is discussed and explored. The model draws on my research and widens its scope to explore its application in EOL care more generally. Also, the context in which the model can be applied and become effective is discussed and explored. The latter topic is extended in the concluding section of the book.

'Conclusions' will draw on the central concepts from this study to offer some concluding thoughts and future trends in practice, policy and research.

Note

1. For more information visit www.ons.gov.uk.

References

Aries, P., 1974. *Western attitudes toward death: From the Middle Ages to the present.* Baltimore, MD: Johns Hopkins University Press.

Becker, E., 1971. *The birth and death of meaning.* New York, NY: Free Press.

Berger, P.L., 1999. The desecularization of the world: A global overview. In Berger, P.L. (ed.), *The desecularization of the world: Resurgent religion and world politics.* Washington, DC: William B. Eerdmans, pp. 1–18.

Bulkley, J., McMullen, C.K., Hornbrok, M.C., Grant, M., Altschuler, A., Wendel, C.S. and Krouse, R.S., 2013. Spiritual well-being in long-term colorectal cancer survivors with ostomies. *Psycho-Oncology*, 22(11), pp. 2513–2521.

Cook, E.L. and Silverman, M.J., 2013. Effects of music therapy on spirituality with patients on a medical oncology/hematology unit: A mixed-methods approach. *The Arts in Psychotherapy*, 40(2), pp. 239–244.

Davie, G., 2013. *The sociology of religion: A critical agenda.* London, UK: Sage.

Davie, G., 2007. Vicarious religion: A methodological challenge. In Ammerman, N.T. (ed.), *Everyday religion: Observing modern religious lives.* New York, NY: Oxford University Press, pp. 21–36.

Davie, G., 1994. *Religion in Britain since 1945: Believing without belonging (making contemporary Britain).* Oxford: Blackwell.

Davies, J., 2013. *Death, burial and rebirth in the religions of antiquity.* London, UK: Routledge.

Department of Health, 2009. *Spiritual care at the end of life: A systematic review of the literature.* London, UK: Department of Health.

Dinham, A., 2015. Religious literacy and welfare. In Dinham, A. and Francis, M. (eds.), *Religious literacy in policy and practice.* Bristol, UK: Policy Press, pp. 101–112.

Dinham, A., 2012. *Faith and social capital after the debt crisis.* Hampshire, UK: Palgrave Macmillan.

Dinham, A. and Francis, M. (eds.), 2015. *Religious literacy in policy and practice.* Bristol: Policy Press.

Doka, K.J., Neimeyer, R.A., Wittkowski, J., Vallerga, M. and Currelley, L., 2016. Productivity in thanatology: An international analysis. *Omega: Journal of Death and Dying*, 73(4), pp. 340–354.

Donnison, D.V., 1980. The discovery and development of knowledge. In International Association of Schools of Social Work (IASSW), *Discovery and development in social work education.* Vienna: IASSW, pp. 11–23.

Edwards, P., Freeman, E. and Sugden, S.J., 1979. *Heidegger on death: A critical evaluation.* La Salle: Hegeler Institute.

Elias, N., 1985. *The loneliness of the dying.* New York, NY: Blackwell.

Emanuel, L.L. and Librach, S.L., 2011. *Palliative care e-book: Core skills and clinical competencies.* St. Louis, MO: Elsevier Health Sciences.

Exline, J.J., Prince-Paul, M., Root, B.L. and Peereboom, K.S., 2013. The spiritual struggle of anger toward God: A study with family members of hospice patients. *Journal of Palliative Medicine.* 16(4), pp. 369–375.

Feifel, H. (ed.), 1959. *The meaning of death.* Maidenhead, UK: McGraw-Hill.

Fonseca, L.M. and Testoni, I., 2011–2012. The emergence of thanatology and current practice in death education. *Omega: Journal of Death and Dying*, 64(2), pp. 157–169.

Freud, S., 1915. Thoughts for the times on war and death. *Standard Edition*, 14(27), pp. 274–302.

Ghesquiere, A.R., Aldridge, M.D., Johnson-Hürzeler, R., Kaplan, D., Bruce, M.L. and Bradley, E., 2015. Hospice services for complicated grief and depression: Results from a national survey. *Journal of the American Geriatrics Society*, 63(10), pp. 2173–2180.

Gijsberts, M.-J.H.E., van der Steen, J.T., Muller, M.T., Hertogh, C.M.P.M. and Deliens, L., 2013. Spiritual end-of-life care in Dutch nursing homes: An ethnographic study. *Journal of the American Medical Directors Association*. 14(9), pp. 679–684.

Gorer, G., 1955. The pornography of death. *Encounter*, 5, pp. 49–52.

Grimes, R.L., Husken, U., Simon, U. and Venbrux, E., 2011. *Ritual, media, and conflict*. Oxford: Oxford University Press.

Healy, D.E., 2013. And what did I do? *Journal of Social Work in End-of-Life & Palliative Care*. 9(2–3), pp. 117–122.

Heidegger, M., 1962. *Seit und Zeit*. 7th ed., Tübingen, Germany: Harper & Row.

Henoch, I., Danielson, E., Strang, S., Browall, M. and Melin-Johansson, C., 2013. Training intervention for health care staff in the provision of existential support to patients with cancer: A randomized, controlled study. *Journal of Pain and Symptom Management*, 46(6), pp. 785–794.

Herbert, M., 1980. Teaching social work in individuals and groups: The knowledge base and impact of research. In International Association of Schools of Social Work (IASSW), *Discovery and development in social work education*. New York, NY: IASSW, pp. 65–69.

Hess, D., 2013. Faith healing and the palliative care team. *Journal of Social Work in End-of-Life & Palliative Care*, 9(2–3), pp. 180–190.

Jewell, A., 2004. *Ageing, spirituality and well-being*. New York, NY: Jessica Kingsley.

Kastenbaum, R.J., 2007. *Death, society, and human experience*, 9th ed., New York, NY: Pearson Education.

Kastenbaum, R., 2000. *The psychology of death*. New York, NY: Springer Publishing.

Kuebler, K.K., Davis, M.P. and Moore, C.D., 2005. *Palliative practices: An interdisciplinary approach*. St Louis, MO: Elsevier Mosby.

Lucchetti, G., Bassi, R.M. and Lucchetti, A.L.G., 2013. Taking spiritual history in clinical practice: A systematic review of instruments. *EXPLORE: The Journal of Science and Healing*, 9(3), pp. 159–170.

McSherry, W. and Ross, L., 2010. *Spiritual assessment in healthcare practice*. Cumbria, UK: M&K Update.

Morin, E., 1951. *L'homme et la mort dans l'histoire [The man and the death in history]*. Paris: Correa.

Nelsen, J.C., 1980. *Communication theory and social work practice*. Monograph collection (Matt – Pseudo). Chicago, IL: University of Chicago Press.

Nelson-Becker, H., 2013. Spirituality in end-of-life and palliative care: What matters? *Journal of Social Work in End-of-Life & Palliative Care*, 9(2–3), pp. 112–116.

Pattison, G., 2013. *Heidegger on death: A critical theological essay*. Washington, DC: Ashgate.

Pentaris, P., 2013. Health care practitioners and dying patients. *Journal of Education, Culture and Society*, 4(1), pp. 38–44.

Public Health England, 2016. Faith at end of life: A resource for professionals, providers and commissioners working in community. Available at: https://www.gov.uk/government/uploads/system/uploads/attachment_data/file/496231/Faith_at_end_of_life_-_a_resource.pdf.

Rogers, C.R., 1979. The foundations of the person-centered approach. *Education,* 100(2), pp. 98–107.

Saunders, D.C., 2005. *Cicely Saunders – Founder of the hospice movement: Selected letters 1959–1999.* Oxford: Oxford University Press.

Stanworth, R., 2004. *Recognizing spiritual needs in people who are dying.* Ann Arbor, MI: Oxford University Press.

Van Baaren, T.P., 1967. Conceptions of life after death. *Bijdragen: International Journal of Philosophy and Theology,* 28(3), pp. 248–259.

Walter, T., 2002. Spirituality in palliative care: Opportunity or burden? *Palliative Medicine,* 16(2), pp. 133–140.

Walter, T., 1994. *The revival of death.* London, UK: Routledge.

Weber, M., 1978. *Economy and society: An outline of interpretive sociology* (Vol.1). Oakland, CA: University of California Press.

Westphal, M., 1984. *God, guilt, and death: An existential phenomenology of religion.* Bloomington, IN: Indiana University Press.

Wilson, B., 1976. *Contemporary transformations of religion.* London, UK: Oxford University Press.

Wilson, B., 1966. *Religion in secular society.* London, UK: C.A. Watts.

Wright, P.M. and Hogan, N.S., 2008. Grief theories and models: Applications to hospice nursing practice. *Journal of Hospice & Palliative Nursing,* 10(6), pp. 350–356.

Part I

Hospice care and changing religious landscape

1 Religion, belief and spirituality in hospice care

Introduction

Amongst the main contemporary scholars who have identified the need for responses to religion, belief and spiritual identities in EOL care are Daaleman and VandeCreek (2000). They hold the view that 'an understanding of religion and spirituality within the context of end of life care, quality of life and patient–clinician interactions may illuminate the problems and potentialities for both patients and clinicians' (Daaleman and VandeCreek, 2000, p. 2514). Nonetheless, the core challenge in this attempt is whether religion and spirituality are perceived as part of the problem or part of the solution. Some examples follow to illustrate this. The approach that Daaleman and VandeCreek followed (2000) had been influenced by the SUPPORT method (Study to Understand Prognoses and Preferences for Outcomes and Risks of Treatment). This method refers to a project beginning in the 1990s which identified, among other things, aspects of religion and belief in the needs of terminally ill patients. The core objective of the study, like that of the HELP Project (Hospitalized Elderly Longitudinal Project), was to address national concerns about patients' freedom to make their own choices when nearing the end of their lives. Furthermore, it sought to reduce the frequency of prolonged, painful and complicated deaths. The SUPPORT project suggests characteristics of care and treatment and highlighted the decision-making patterns of critically ill patients (Daaleman and VandeCreek, 2000), whereas this book's argument goes beyond those aspects of care, promoting a redressing of the balance in the relationship amongst hospice care, religion, belief and spirituality. These are valuable aspects of EOL care:

> The goal of a quality comfortable death is achieved by meeting a patient's physical needs and by attending to the social, psychological, and the now recognized spiritual and religious dimensions of care (Daaleman and VandeCreek, 2000, p. 2514).

This approach of quality care to institutional dying (Stevenson et al., 2007) recalls previous examples regarding the enhancement and enrichment of healthcare more generally. One example is found in the United States. In the late 1980s, a consensus statement included the embedding of the religious and spiritual needs of patients in healthcare; however, it referred to them as problems: 'assess and manage psychological, social, and spiritual/ religious problems' (Cassel and Foley, 1999, p. 6). An additional remark regarding the approach informed by this quote is that it had reinforced the management of 'religious and spiritual problems as core principles of professional practice and care at end of life' (Daaleman and VandeCreek, 2000, p. 2514). This attitude has significantly informed death policies (also discussed in Chapter 3), as well as attitudes towards spirituality in EOL care. An example of the latter is Daaleman et al. (2008); in their explanatory study of nursing homes, they conclude that nurses and doctors believe that the spiritual and religious needs of their patients are merely fluid processes of their personal development towards the end of their lives. Outside the institutional context of a hospice, or home for the elderly, and beyond their social and collective dimensions (Smart, 1996), religion and belief are matters subject to individual consciousness. This seems to be overtly challenging to hospice professionals in institutional care, perhaps due to lack of confidence in engaging with aspects of care over which one may not have authority (Yardley, Walshe and Parr, 2009). For example, physicians would monitor and audit pain management but would find themselves professionally vulnerable in the face of needs that derive from spiritual suffering. This is not to suggest all hospice professionals share the same vulnerabilities, but to emphasise the logic behind professional uncertainty surrounding religious and spiritual needs.

Another example worth noting is the UK End of Life Care Strategy 2008, which highlights spiritual needs but not religious ones, with the former being bracketed in the Strategy with requirements for the meeting of emotional needs. This is addressed neither in the NHS Improving Quality (guidelines for improving healthcare) nor in professional practise. In other words, spiritual care is included in the principal responsibilities of hospice professionals, as it is an integral part of the holistic care the NHS has striven to offer (Department of Health, 2003). This was predicted by Walter in the 1990s, writing that 'spiritual care will become indistinguishable in practice from emotional/psychological care' (Walter, 1997, p. 29). His prognosis has come true to a wide extent, as the example of the End of Life Care Strategy reveals.

These examples not only emphasise the requirement for care inclusive of all aspects of an individual's needs, but also show the unclear understanding of the terms 'religion', 'belief', 'spirituality', or of other terms (e.g. 'faith') used to discuss spiritual care. One of the most challenging moments in this context is the minimal recognition of non-religion and non-belief – concepts that do not come without challenge. Lee (2012), for example, identified the definitional issues faced in the ever-growing field of nonreligion, and recommended a working definition, which separates secularity, secularism and atheism, to assist scholars and researchers from across disciplines. Whether this suggestion is effective is, however, debatable (Guyau, 2015). In other words, the problem with the concepts of nonreligion or nonbelief is the same as with terms like 'religion', 'belief', 'faith' or 'spirituality': There is no clear definition that can adequately describe what these concepts entail. Rather, they are each redefined each time they are used in literature.

Equally important is the ambiguity among the terms 'religion', 'belief', 'faith' and 'spirituality'. Scholars have supported various ideas concerning the meaning and content of each concept, yet practises and policies reflect their complicated nature. Regardless of previous works, this book focusses on exploring the concept of belief, whether religious or nonreligious. In doing so, it refers to religion, belief and spirituality as an inclusive cluster of all variations of people's identified faith or lack thereof. There is emphasis in this chapter and throughout the book on the tense relationship between spirituality and religion. The former is more acknowledged whereas the latter has lacked clear recognition during past decades (Davie, 2015), for reasons explained in Chapter 2.

The literature largely confines itself to discussions of spirituality, whereas religion and belief are continuously marginalised. This undermines the demand for engagement with religion, belief and spiritual identities, and suggests that, in any case, talk of spirituality does not signify commitment in practise. Having said this, it would be unfair to undermine the latest attempts made in hospice care to address religion by name, although attempts have followed a linear approach aiming to increase knowledge about different religious traditions. An example of that in the UK is the document *Faith at the end of life*, released by Public Health England (PHE) in 2016. This is a resource for professionals as well as for commissioners and providers of end of life care in the community. The resource focusses on highlighting the shifting demographics of religious identity in the UK, but identifies only a few predominant religious profiles, such as Christianity, discussing the practises and beliefs of that particular religion about death and dying.

Despite all recent attempts to increase factual knowledge about various religious views and practises about death and dying, discourses about service users and their psychosocial needs remain centred around spirituality. However, this comes with an increasing challenge; many scholars affirm spirituality to be a contested notion. In his view, Walter (2002) suggests alternative approaches and challenges an assumption in palliative care literature – namely, the claim that all patients have spiritual needs and that palliative professionals have the right skills and knowledge to provide spiritual care.

> If all patients have spiritual needs, if the palliative care unit is committed to holistic care, and if all members of the multi-disciplinary team can deliver this kind of spiritual care, logic then requires that they ought to deliver it. (Walter, 2002, p. 3)

Research on spirituality (Puchalski, 2013; Ferrell, Otis-Green and Economou, 2013), however, shows that spirituality has not been successfully integrated into in-patient or out-patient hospice services, nor has it found its ethical embedment in the professional lives of hospice members of staff, at least not evidently. Spiritual care is often described as addressing a wide range of needs, from emotional to social and religious, but with little specifications of its limits. An undeniable disciplinary challenge is present; on the one hand, social workers have largely offered psychosocial and emotional support, even before its recognition as a profession (Ehrenreich, 2014; Healy, 2008; Austin, 1983), and not only in hospice care. On the other hand, both chaplains (Nolan, 2012) and nurses (McSherry, 1998) have, by and large, contributed to the delivery of spiritual care in contemporary practise and claimed further disciplinary responsibility. The consensus here is an ongoing debate about disciplinary boundaries, which seem blurred, and which impact on the quality and consistency of hospice services. However, this is not the only challenge identified in the discourses about spiritual care.

Wynne (2013, abstract) claims that 'there is a lack of awareness of the importance of spirituality in patients' lives, and how competent spiritual care can enhance quality of life and improve patient outcomes'. Equally, Puchalski (2013) suggests that there is a lack of understanding of what spirituality in hospice care entails. My argument reflects the spectrum of religion, belief and spirituality in the religious landscape according to the social scientific evidence, whereas policy confines itself predominantly to discussions of spirituality. This leaves religion and belief as neglected aspects of identity or identities in hospice care. Consequently, the marginalisation of religion and belief in hospice care is thought to be supported by the experiences of dying people themselves (Pentaris, 2018). Religion and belief are, by nature, unmeasurable and inconsistent with the mechanical and bureaucratic tendencies of care. Therefore, it is to some extent logical that the achievement-based approach to EOL care is challenged when asked to incorporate those aspects of need into care delivery. This is the result of the ongoing progression of approaches to caring for the dying and bereaved with biomedical and clinical approaches taking hold in contemporary hospice practise.

Biomedical and clinical approaches are taking hold in EOL care (Hollins, 2006; also see Paley, 2008, for jurisdictions of care in hospices), which poses the challenge of how to integrate religion, belief and spiritual identities of service users in policy and practise. Since the development of the hospice movement in the late 1960s, EOL care has seen numerous challenges in a fast-changing society, with its shifting composition, complications and contested notions. So, according to Daaleman et al. (2008), multiple ethical and pragmatic issues emerge from the conversation regarding integrating religion, belief and spiritual needs into healthcare in general, and in EOL care in particular. 'Should physicians identify patients' spiritual and religious needs and intervene in clinical settings?' (Daaleman and VandeCreek, 2000, p. 2514). This is a key question that could apply to all healthcare professions as well as allied professions in the sector. This was also noted by Puchalski et al. (2006, p. 398), who claim that 'in order to provide excellent palliative care physicians and other healthcare professionals must be able to address all these dimensions of care [physical, emotional and social], including the spiritual'.

This book's arguments go beyond identifying needs and appointing professional responsibilities. Since Saunders' perception of spiritual care in hospices (Saunders, 1988), and including the recent review of the emergence of spiritual dimensions in EOL care in the UK in 2011 by the Department of Health (DH), the discussion and intentions remain the same. Saunders initiated the dialogue about spirituality, and this has surfaced and resurfaced ever since in a variety of policies and guidance. However, the conversation appears not to have matured or evolved in keeping with developments in the understanding of the sociology of religion. Specifically, religion, belief and spirituality are not well understood and are even less well operationalised.

Hospice movement

It is impossible to talk about religion, belief and spiritual identities of service users in hospice care without reviewing the history and development of the hospice movement. It would also be unorthodox to set out to explore professionals' attitudes to and experiences of delivering care regarding these identities without first properly introducing the context in which this takes place. Before I embark with this task, however, it is worth noting that whilst the vision of hospice care has travelled across the globe over the decades, the current account focusses only on the development of hospice care in the UK, with occasional references to the US, as the UK is the social context that has been the main canvas for the study that informs this book.

The past nearly 60 years have seen improvements in the care afforded to the terminally ill and in pain management. Medical research in symptomatology has expanded and new treatments have emerged for pain control. Simultaneously, scholars from sociology and psychology have further developed their interest in death studies and provided critical thinking that 'has reshaped contemporary views of death' (Forman et al., 2003, p. 1). An example of the latter is Philippe Aries, whose work was influenced by Gorer's (1955) argument about the pornography of death. Aries (1974) explored western attitudes to death and suggests that death was as concealed a matter in the 20th century as sexuality was in the 19th. Another example includes Herman Feifel (1959), whose work not only influenced professional practise with patients with terminal illnesses, but also inspired Cicely Saunders, one of the key figures in the development of hospice care. Despite all the achievements until the third quarter of the 20th, 'it was the work of two physicians, Elisabeth Kübler-Ross and Dame Cicely Saunders ... that began to change the way society and health professionals perceived terminal disease, death, and dying' (Forman et al., 2003, pp. 1–2).

Cicely Saunders is renowned for her work with patients with terminal illnesses. She is also acclaimed as a pioneer of modern hospice care. She set out in the late 1940s to contribute in this area with a clear vision in mind, and her work has since influenced systems of care for the dying across the world (Clark, 2002). It is in that vision one can locate the beginning of the modern history of hospice care.

Amongst those who have reviewed Saunders' work is Clark (2002). He provides a neutral account that lays out the progression of Saunders's thinking while conceiving her vision of hospice care. Clark's work introduces a considerable amount of the correspondence sent by Saunders to numerous colleagues, friends, and members of the Church since she began envisioning changes in the care of the dying, and continuing up until the early 1990s. At this point, St. Christopher's Hospice had already become the beacon of care for the dying, and palliative care was taking hold in policy and education (Clark, 2002).

Cicely Saunders was British and a highly devout Christian with a strong and firm affiliation to the Church of England. According to Clark (2002), she felt a special connection to God. She was a qualified nurse, who had also practised as an almoner. Due to her keen interest in caring for patients with terminal cancer, she undertook medical education and qualified as a medical doctor in her late 30s. She was to become one of the first modern doctors with a special interest in EOL care – an area that had previously seen scant attention.

Her vision becomes clear from her very first publication in the *St. Thomas's Hospital Gazette* in 1958, in which she argued for new approaches to the care of the dying:

> Many patients feel deserted by their doctors at the end. Ideally the doctor should remain the centre of a team who work together to relieve where they cannot heal, to keep the patient's own struggle within the compass and to bring hope and consolation to the end. (Saunders, 1958, p. 46)

The vision was clear; the new approach would aim to care for dying people, easing suffering and pain when treatment was not available. This was imagined as a task for a whole team and not for individual professionals. Saunders spent some years volunteering for the St. Joseph's Hospice in Hackney, London, where her ideas of how to pursue this teamwork approach were informed. These experiences helped her to grasp the purpose of a team of healthcare and allied professionals that together provide support in alleviating the *total pain* of the patients (Clark, 1999), a concept discussed later in this chapter.

Across a span of approximately 15 years, Saunders sought advice and guidance from many people from both sides of the Atlantic. Much of her influence came from nuns from the Irish Sisters of Charity at St. Joseph's Hospice, psychologist Herman Feifel, psychiatrist Colin Murray Parkes, evangelical Christian lawyer Jack Wallace, and theologian Olive Wyon, to name a few. Yet, her biggest influence in setting out to explore the idea of caring for the dying was her own religious faith, practised in the Church of England. Drawing from one of her letters, dated 9 February 1960, as published by Clark (2002, p. 20), Saunders writes to the Lord Bishop of Stepney: 'I am very anxious that this work should be a Church of England one, and that it should be broadly based in the Church'. There are numerous examples that suggest that Saunders acted as a Christian believer when approaching EOL care (Clark, 2002; Clark and Seymour, 1999; du Boulay, 2007). Her Christian beliefs became paramount in the development of St Christopher's Hospice in the late 1960s, the physical space in which her vision would come true. By that time, the NHS was involved in supporting this initiative, despite it being a newly established one.

The commencement of service provision at St. Christopher's Hospice in 1967 was led by the following principles:

- Death must be accepted;
- The patient's total care must be managed by a skilled interdisciplinary team whose members communicate regularly with one another;
- The common symptoms of terminal disease, especially the palliation of pain in all its aspects, need to be effectively controlled;
- The patient and family must be recognised as a single unit of care;
- An active home-care programme should be implemented;
- An active programme of bereavement care for the family after the death of the patient must be provided;
- Research and education should be ongoing (Forman et al., 2003, p. 5; revised from Torrens, 1985).

In the same period, Elisabeth Kübler-Ross was striving to introduce to the public and professionals the very first framework through which the stages of the experience of dying would be operationalised. Even though Bowlby's work in the late 1940s on attachment and loss was already adding to the conversation, it was not explicitly turned into guidance for professional practitioners. Kübler-Ross, having interviewed dying patients, published *On Death and Dying* in 1969. With this book, and her now popular five-stage model of grief (its critiques notwithstanding) (Parkes, 2013), Kübler-Ross managed to breach the public silence around the subject of death and dying. Her arguments travelled across the world, and her work influenced and still influences professional practise in many nations. Kübler-Ross' work also opened up space for more robust initiatives in the US, following the work of Cicely Saunders, including hospices and palliative care units within hospitals (Clark and Seymour, 1999).

There is one paradox worth noting in the history of the hospice movement in the UK. This is most clearly described by Clark and Seymour (1999, p. 69):

> One of the paradoxes of the history of the modern hospice movement in Britain is that it was to originate in the shadow of a new, inclusive

system of socialized medicine and welfare which would care for all in need, 'from the cradle to the grave' .... Like the voluntary hospices which had preceded it, however, the priorities of the British National Health Service ... were with acute illness and rehabilitation. This, coupled with an ideological rejection of charity as the appropriate source for the provision of health care, did not create an auspicious environment in which voluntary hospices might be expected to develop.

Also worth mentioning is that the terms 'hospice movement' and 'palliative care' were not used until the 1970s (Forman et al., 2003). By the beginning of the 21st century, there were numerous hospices and palliative care units across the globe, including examples in Australia, New Zealand, Western Europe, Eastern Europe, Asia and North America. The World Health Organization (WHO) recognised the importance of the concept and emphasised the attention it was giving to clearing the definitional boundaries. A clear-cut definition of palliative care was offered which would incorporate all aspects of a patient's needs:

> Palliative care is the active, total care of patients whose disease is not responsive to curative treatment. Control of pain, other symptoms, and of psychological, social and spiritual problems is paramount. The goal of palliative care is achievement of the best possible quality of life for patients and their families. Many aspects of palliative care are also applicable earlier in the course of illness, in conjunction with anti-cancer treatment. (Forman et al., 2003, p. 8)

This definition has changed a few times over the years, however, and its current form is as follows:

> Palliative care is an approach that improves the quality of life of patients and their families facing the problem associated with life-threatening illness, through the prevention and relief of suffering by means of early identification and impeccable assessment and treatment of pain and other problems, physical, psychosocial and spiritual. (WHO, 2012)

Despite the disparities in the two versions, which date approximately 15 years apart, both imply a multi-dimensional patient and put emphasis on multidisciplinary practise. Also, in spite of the identification of the patients' needs as problems which pose different challenges, both definitions recognise spirituality and the professional need to attend to that aspect of the patient's care. It is that aspect of hospice care that this book explores; however, it broadens its scope to address the religious, belief and spiritual identities of service users all together, and not spirituality in isolation.

The following two sub-sections explore the term 'total pain', that has led the development of the principles of hospice care into their current form

(Clark and Seymour, 1999), and the interdisciplinary approach that contemporary hospice care emphasises (Saunders, 1991; Eustler and Martinez, 2003). This leads to an exploration of the presence and absence of spirituality, religion and belief in hospice care.

'Total pain'

'Total pain' is a term coined by Cicely Saunders in the 1960s. Informed by the stories she had been hearing from her patients at St. Joseph's Hospice since the late 1950s, she developed the concept of total pain to introduce the multi-faceted character of pain as patients experience it:

> By the time that Cicely Saunders left St. Joseph's in 1965, she had collected detailed descriptions of the cases of 1,100 patients, and there was clear evidence of a sustained and determined attempt to understand pain as a multidimensional phenomenon in which physical and mental suffering were inseparable, and in which pain relief required something more than mere attention to medical treatments. (Seymour, Clark and Winslow, 2005, p. 9)

There are four components to this formulation: physical, mental, spiritual and emotional/social suffering (Seymour, Clark and Winslow, 2005). Saunders' understanding of total pain, Clark (2000, abstract) claims, was the product of her own professional background as a nurse, almoner and physician: 'it emerged from Cicely Saunders' unique experience as nurse, social worker, and physician – the remarkable multidisciplinary platform from which she launched the hospice movement'. According to Saunders (1996), total pain is also a process, during which people reflect on their lives, and in turn causes multiple types of suffering.

Saunders (2001) recognised the importance of allowing the patient to be involved in defining their own suffering, whilst professionals advocate a holistic approach to that suffering, regardless of its particularity (also see Clark, 1999). In other words, the development of the concept of total pain, made the need for an interdisciplinary approach as pertinent as it was pressing (Bonica, 1953; Clark, 1999).

Interdisciplinary team

Some 20 years after the establishment of St. Christopher's Hospice, Saunders (1990) wrote about her ideal of an interdisciplinary approach to hospice and palliative care. She did this through impressionistic metaphors in which patients are surrounded by their home, their work and other aspects of their lives. 'It is this scene that we are addressing …. We are a collage comprised of all the different professions involved in the total care of the person who is approaching death' (Saunders, 1990, p. v).

In its modern history, the healthcare system is characterised by holistic care, which in turn has adopted an interdisciplinary approach 'for addressing patients' complex healthcare needs (Eustler and Martinez 2003, p. 13). Eustler and Martinez (2003) argue that each profession and discipline has a different set of knowledge and skills to contribute to the care of the dying. Similarly, Puchalski et al. (2006, p. 398) suggest that 'physicians and other healthcare professionals must be able to address all these dimensions of care, including the spiritual'. An example of how this works in practise is given by Howard (2001), who explicitly identifies the different dimensions of the total pain of a patient, and thereafter links each part to the discipline that could ease that pain.

According to Eustler and Martinez (2003, p. 13), 'the goal of the interdisciplinary team is to work with patients to identify their specific needs and health goals within a holistic framework'. Each member of the team contributes in a unique way and supports the alleviation of the suffering of the patient, and this has been central to hospice care since the inception of its vision (Clark, 1999).

The previous subsections have introduced the history and development of the hospice movement, as well as highlighting two central concepts in hospice and palliative care: those of total pain and the interdisciplinary approach. In other words, we now have a platform (hospice care) with certain characteristics (total pain and the interdisciplinary approach) in which the discussion about spiritual care can develop.

Spirituality and hospice care

It is clear by now that one of hospice care's main dimensions is detailed attention to spiritual needs, with the intention being to alleviate spiritual pain and suffering. This is a very different concept to physical pain, when administration of the appropriate drugs can make all the difference. How does one go about relieving someone from spiritual pain? Many proposed answers are available in scholarly works, and although some are discussed later, it is worth noting here the following, as starting points. Both Saunders (1990, 1988) and Kübler-Ross (1969) suggested that listening to patients is the essential act in providing spiritual comfort – and comfort in general. Beyond their bio-physical symptoms and needs, patients want to have their feelings and emotions heard, and have the opportunity to discuss existential issues with their healthcare giver, who is often a nurse (McSherry, 2001). Spiritual care provision is time-consuming and requires intensive engagement; these are two aspects of promoting care to which we return in Parts II and III of this book.

Until the late 1980s, the spiritual dimension of hospice care made reference to Christianity only (du Boulay, 2007). The Church of England played a critical role in the development and formation of hospice care; Saunders, according to her own letters, had been guided by God to undertake this task (Clark, 1999). Saunders (1988) introduced Christian concepts and made them central to her work. She referred to the Bible in her writings and recognised St. Christopher's Hospice as a Christian Institution:

> The Christian and medical foundation of St. Christopher's was concerned with the response to these costly demands, as it set out in the belief that God would provide both people and resources if we worked the plan out in the right way. We believed that in this response we would learn to be the instruments of His care for the suffering and bereaved, and show our patients and their families the care by deeds rather than words which would help them into a healing relationship with Him and also help to encourage new skills and attitudes far more widely. (Saunders, 1986, cited in Saunders, 2006, p. 42)

It is appropriate to consider how this Christian framework has influenced the hospice movement. Excellent examples are the names of hospices across the UK, such as St. Luke's Hospice or St. Ann's Hospice. Another example of how Christian beliefs have been present in the development and formation of hospices is the frequent contribution of nuns. Both examples show the focus on Christianity and the lack of inter-faith approaches in EOL care that persisted until recent years.

Despite her highly Christian devotion and influence, Saunders was of the view that all patients and staff should have the opportunity for spiritual growth, regardless of their faith, belief, or nonbelief:

> We are ourselves a community of the unlike, coming from different faiths and denominations or the absence of any commitment of this kind. What we have in common is concern of each individual ... and our hope is that each person will think as deeply as he can in his own way. (Saunders, 2006, cited in Coward and Stajduhar, 2012, p. 3)

Spiritual care is critical in contemporary practise in EOL care and most relevant to scholarly work across different disciplines. Spiritual care is contested in its definition, as is the definition of its counterpart and instigator: spiritual need. Saunders defines spiritual needs as follows:

> 'Spiritual' concerns the spirit or higher moral qualities, especially as regarded in a religious aspect with beliefs and practises held to more or less faithfully. But 'spiritual' also covers much more than that – the meaning of life at its deepest levels as understood through our patients' different religions. (Saunders, 1988, p. 218)

Saunders continues, delineating the concept of 'spiritual pain':

> The realization that life is likely to end soon may well stimulate a desire to put first things first and to reach out to what is seen as true and

valuable – and give rise to feelings of being unable or unworthy to do so. There may be bitter anger at the unfairness of what is happening, and at much of what has gone before, and above all a desolate feeling of meaningless. Herein lies, I believe, the essence of spiritual pain. (Saunders, 1988, p. 218)

Being well enough equipped to identify spiritual needs and pain, also raises another challenge: identifying the appropriate care for those needs, or having the willingness to do so.

The spiritual dimension of modern hospice care

There has been increasing concern since the mid 1990s that the original hospice ethos is reforming and becoming subject to secularity and bureaucratisation (Bradshaw, 1996; Clark and Seymour, 1999). This change is evident in the care that hospices provide, as well as in the profile of carers.

> The story of the changes in care for the chronic sick and terminally ill is also the story of the changes in nursing from altruism and service to the patient, derived from a spiritual ethic, to empowerment and liberation for nursing, derived from a concern with professional autonomy. It is the story of the twentieth century secularisation of care. The changed ethic of care runs deeply throughout the care services ... and has obviously affected the ethos of hospice care. (Bradshaw, 1996, p. 410).

Bradshaw (1996) explored the 'routinisation' thesis to argue that from a hospice system of care, where a 'spiritual calling' was essential for the professionals (also see du Boulay, 2007), the secularisation thesis has led to 'an iron cage' of duty (Bradshaw, 1996, p. 409). In other words, Bradshaw scrutinises the spiritual dimension of hospice care to find that 'traditional, orthodox spirituality, the human being in relationship to God, has been replaced by a conception of spirituality as a personal and psychological search for meaning' (Bradshaw, 1996, p. 416) (also see James and Field, 1992). She also argued that Saunders 'was reviving an attitude to death as part of life at a time in the twentieth century when Aries argues, the desire was to hide death away' (Bradshaw, 1996, p. 413; also see Aries, 1974). Until the 20th century, death had been more routinely encountered during the 20th and into the 21st centuries. However, public attitudes saw death as a weakness. Considering such belief, medical approaches to the prolonging of life became more important than embracing the full circle of life, which would have been a more spiritual approach to take.

Spiritual need in 21st-century hospice care must necessarily be considered differently than it was in the 1960s and 1970s. However, the care of the dying and the bereaved has always had a connection with religion; Bradshaw examined the changes to this over time. Death is no longer happening in the home (Walter, 1997, 1999; Bradshaw, 1996). In fact, 'two-thirds of all deaths today take place in hospital – an institution dominated by science and medicine' (Walter, 1997, p. 22). This creates further challenges in integrating spiritual care in practise, mostly stemming from the division between science and religion/spirituality, especially after the shift from *terminal care* to *palliative care*:

> The shift from terminal care to the much wider area of palliative care is a shift in emphasis which alters the original concept of improving care of dying people. Palliative care shifts the focus of attention away from death and there is a real danger that by talking about focusing upon palliation, people may stop talking about and confronting the fact that the individual is going to die. (Biswas, 1993, p. 135)

Walter (1997) subjects spiritual care to extensive scrutiny. His work is concerned with what spiritual care might mean today and how that might fit into a highly secular context. He examines three options through which spiritual care might find a peaceful place in the context of the highly bureaucratic, secular and institutionalised hospice care of today.

Drawing from Christianity's principal concerns about death (i.e., 'love of the neighbour and concern for the post-mortem destination of the human soul' [Walter, 1997, p. 22]), Walter introduces the hospice as a religious community. Both Bradshaw (1996) and Walter (1997) raise the point that spirituality may be the concern only of religious staff members in a hospice. What happens, though, when 'secular' staff are hired to deliver hospice care? Both Bradshaw and Walter argue that such expansion of care causes conflict and tension, which may undermine quality of care for the dying. If we accept that spiritual care can only be delivered by religious staff members, we are also challenging the concept of holistic care, as discussed earlier, and its call for an interdisciplinary approach and the care of the whole person by recognising their total pain. As Walter (1997) suggests, if spiritual care is enabled only by the *charisma* and *discernment* of religious people, there may be major deficits in the provision of spiritual care for many dying people outside hospices and within the contemporary secular and technocratic formation of hospice care (Clark and Seymour, 1999). The following quote renders this in Walter's words:

> How is this gift [gift of discernment], this charisma, to be routinized in the larger and more bureaucratic institutions that hospices may turn into, or in the large hospitals that hospices aim to influence? Can thousands be expected to have this gift? If not, can such a gift be taught? If all nurses are expected to provide spiritual care, how may those without this particular gift or indeed without religious commitment discern when a patient is raising spiritual issues and know how to respond? (Walter, 1997, p. 24)

The first option seems problematic in a number of ways, including a different stance on, and very different definition of, spirituality, from what Saunders intended. Furthermore, with the second option, Walter's argument is straightforward; if this is the option preferred, then spiritual care should naturally find a place under the jurisdiction of members of staff who are clergy or other religious leaders. Clark and Seymour (1999, p. 110) claim that 'spiritual is the same as religious; only some people are religious; non-religious and non-ordained staff are not competent to deal with spiritual needs' while Walter refers to 'calling in the chaplain'. Perhaps this approach is what Nolan (2012) is arguing for; however, he neglects to consider that in letting all other staff members focus on their own remit of practise, while chaplains undertake spiritual care, the idea of true holistic care would be compromised. Perhaps this is a question of what spiritual care actually means, and who should be responsible for its delivery. Nursing literature has widely argued that spiritual care is the responsibility of nurses (Carroll, 2001; McSherry and Draper, 1998; Ross, 2006; Paley, 2008). Nevertheless, current practise has this dimension of hospice care as being the primary responsibility of chaplains. The main disadvantage of this approach, as argued by Walter (1997, p. 25), is that 'it implies that only some patients have a spiritual dimension, and is therefore incompatible with holistic care'.

The third approach identified by Walter appears to reunite holistic care with spirituality:

> This identifies the spiritual with the search for meaning and has more to do with the human spirit as the animating or vital principle in a person – the 'breath of life' – than with religion, narrowly defined. (Walter, 1997, p. 25)

Previous literature has shown that few patients are highly religious (Simsen, 1986). However, a clear majority have spiritual concerns, and therefore have existential questions to be answered towards the end of their lives (Simsen, 1986). Walter revisits Saunders' intentions (i.e. to provide care for all, regardless of religion) and highlights that this option is most likely to meet these foundational objectives of hospice care, and to minimise the risk of the institutionalisation of spiritual care.

This approach also contests the notion that spiritual care is the sole responsibility of one or two professions or disciplines. As mentioned earlier, Nolan (2012) argued that it is the chaplains who should be providing such care, whereas other literature, and notably James and Field (1996) and McSherry, Cash and Ross (2004), claim that nurses should be the ones delivering spiritual care. I, however, do not argue that one professional should be more responsible than another, or advocate for one discipline predominating. The thesis of this volume draws from Walter's (1997) third approach and builds on the argument that all healthcare staff should be well-equipped to address religion, belief and the spiritual needs of the dying and the bereaved. Walter, in particular, suggests this:

> In this third approach, spiritual care becomes the joint responsibility of all members of the multidisciplinary team. Any staff member can listen to patients and help them identify and articulate what is important to them personally. Indeed, a patient may select a nurse or aide who is not him or herself ordained or even overtly religious with whom to discuss existential issues. (Walter, 1997, p. 25)

Literature of the 21st century, by and large, reflects aspects of the medicalisation thesis (Kennedy and Kennedy, 2014), that links to the idea of jurisdictional areas for practise in hospices (Paley, 2008).

Twenty years after Walter's analysis, the hospice and palliative care sectors appear to have embraced a mix of the three options. Gordon and Mitchell (2004) claim that the Marie Curie model of spiritual and religious competencies is critical, and would only benefit professionals if it were to be applied across hospices. The model presents four levels of competency and classifies professionals in each level by their discipline. For example, level 4, the highest, consists of chaplains and other religious leaders (Walter's second approach). This assumes that no other professionals but religious leaders and chaplains could attain a level 4 competency. Furthermore, the classification of competencies presumes the patient and family's spiritual needs can also be classified from high to low.

On the other hand, Kellehear (2000) suggests a theoretical model of needs. He identifies three blocks of needs within the spiritual dimension: situational, moral and biographical, and religious. This model may also be an outline of the different ways in which spiritual care can be delivered. It also seems to be a new perspective on the interdisciplinary approach, in which where each professional delivers the aspect of spiritual care they feel most comfortable with or are most knowledgeable about.

In their report, Puchalski et al. (2009, p. 885) summarised:

> The need for a commonly accepted definition of spirituality, the appropriate application of spiritual care in palliative care settings, clarification about who should deliver spiritual care, the role of health care providers in spiritual care, and ways to increase scientific rigor surrounding spirituality and spiritual care research and practice.

First, spirituality was identified as 'the aspect of humanity that refers to the way individuals seek and express meaning and purpose and the way they experience their connectedness to the moment, to self, to others, to nature, and to the significant or sacred' (Puchalski et al., 2009, p. 887). This is a definition that most likely aligns with Walter's (1997) suggestion of a 'searching for meaning' approach. It openly invites all members of a team to be the deliverers of spiritual care. Nevertheless, as we move through the report (Puchalski et al., 2009), more technocratic and goal-oriented approaches seem to have dominated the writers' views of hospice care. The following are a few examples.

Engel (1977) and White, Williams and Greenberg (1961) proposed a biomedical model that includes spiritual care. Despite the intention to embrace a focus on the being-in-relationship concept of the individual (Puchalski et al., 2009, pp. 890–891), it is suggested that each aspect (i.e. biological, psychological and social) of the illness is informed by the spiritual. Nevertheless, the medical aspect of the illness drives the need for the spiritual to begin with (White, Williams and Greenberg, 1961). This causes confusion and misunderstandings as to whether the illness is seen through the lens of a patient's beliefs, religious or not.

Furthermore, Puchalski et al. (2009) report on the general suggestions made at the Consensus Conference regarding spiritual care: that spiritual assessment is fundamental to meet the needs of individual patients. So how did hospice professionals at the conference suggest this be done?

> Spiritual screening or triage is a quick determination of whether a person is experiencing a serious spiritual crisis and therefore needs an immediate referral to a board-certified chaplain. Spiritual screening helps identify which patients may benefit from an in-depth spiritual assessment. Good models of spiritual screening use a few simple questions that can be asked in the course of an overall patient and family screening. Examples of such questions include, 'Are spirituality or religion important in your life?' and 'How well are those resources working for you at this time?' (Puchalski et al., 2009, pp. 891 and 893)

This method draws from all three approaches identified by Walter (1997). First, a full screening of spiritual needs requires a 'board-certified chaplain' who provides care of the dying; a religious leader will support religious or spiritual needs (first approach in Walter). So, who is a board-certified chaplain and what is their role? Undeniably, this is a model that induces the 'calling in the chaplain' approach (option 2 in Walter). However, it is acceptable that any member of staff may ask the initial questions which will identify a spiritual crisis (option 3 in Walter) before asking a chaplain to undertake a full spiritual assessment.

In summary

The aforementioned examples are critical of the current approaches to spiritual care in EOL care. However, it would be wrong to examine these examples outside of the policy context that informs, and often dictates, the different ways in which care is delivered. Before we move on to the next two chapters, that address religion and policy more extensively, it is worth recapturing the core themes from the discussion about hospice care and spirituality that have informed the research behind this book.

Hospice care has its roots in religion, most notably Christianity. The care of the dying has been undertaken extensively by religious people in the past (e.g. the Sisters of Ireland), and Saunders' vision did not deviate from this (Saunders, 1958, 2001). The concept of *total pain* emerged to educate professionals and policy-makers about the different dimensions of care necessary for the dying and bereaved. Spirituality was one of those dimensions – the term being used to refer to any belief system. Spiritual care was an essential element of hospice care, which was further developed in the 21st century.

The delivery of spiritual care has caused distress and tension within hospices (also see Cobb, 2001). It causes the blurring of professional responsibilities, as its delivery still lacks clarity. Second, spiritual care raises ethical concerns that are incompatible with the modern bio-medical approaches or methods through which it is understood (Carroll, 2001). In practise, the need for measurable outcomes and results becomes imperative, and this may undermine the importance of respecting a person's religion, belief or spiritual identity (Pentaris, 2014).

An interdisciplinary approach that complements holistic care is pertinent to hospices (McPeak, 2003), but poses several challenges for professionals. The main challenges are identified by Yardley, Walshe and Parr (2009, p. 601) who suggest that 'there are difficulties encountered in delivering optimal spiritual care: first, uncertainty about who should deliver spiritual care; second, lack of confidence and competence in delivering spiritual care in palliative settings and third, difficulty identifying specific spiritual needs'.

The information presented in this volume goes beyond the identification of those challenges in professional practise. It suggests that all hospice professionals should be prepared to support the dying and the bereaved regarding their religion, belief and spiritual identities. Concurrently, it examines the current practises, skills, knowledge and understanding that professionals demonstrate in this area, widening the space for recommendations and the discovery of future trends.

References

Aries, P., 1974. *Western attitudes toward death: From the Middle Ages to the present.* Baltimore, MD: Johns Hopkins University Press.

Austin, D.M., 1983. The Flexner myth and the history of social work. *Social Service Review*, 57(3), pp. 357–377.

Biswas, B., 1993. The medicalisation of dying: A nurse's view. In Clark, D. (ed.), *The future for palliative care: Issues in policy and practice.* Buckingham, UK: Open University Press, pp. 133–139.

Bonica, J.J., 1953. *The management of pain: With special emphasis on the use of analgesic block in diagnosis, prognosis and therapy.* London, UK: Henry Kimpton.

Bradshaw, A., 1996. The spiritual dimension of hospice: The secularization of an ideal. *Social Science Medicine*, 43(3), pp. 409–419.

Carroll, B., 2001. A phenomenological exploration of the nature of spirituality and spiritual care. *Mortality*, 6(1), pp. 81–98.

Cassel, C. and Foley, K.M., 1999. *Principles for care of patients at the end of life: An emerging consensus among the specialties of medicine*. New York, NY: Milbank Memorial Fund.

Clark, D., 2002. *Cicely Saunders: Founder of the hospice movement: Selected letters 1959–1999*. Oxford, UK: Clarendon Press.

Clark, D., 2000. Total pain: The work of Cicely Saunders and the hospice movement. *American Pain Society Bulletin*, 10(4), pp. 13–15.

Clark, D., 1999. Cradled to the grave? Terminal care in the United Kingdom, 1946–1967. *Mortality*, 4(3), pp. 225–247.

Clark, D. and Seymour, J., 1999. *Reflections on palliative care*. Buckingham, UK: Open University Press.

Cobb, M., 2001. *The dying soul: Spiritual care at the end of life*. London, UK: McGraw-Hill Education.

Coward, H. and Stajduhar, K.I. (eds.), 2012. *Religious understandings of a good death in hospice palliative care*. Albany, NY: State University of New York Press.

Daaleman, T.P. and VandeCreek, L., 2000. Placing religion and spirituality in end-of-life care. *Journal of the American Medical Association*, 284(19), pp. 2514–2517.

Daaleman, T.P., Williams, C.S., Hamilton, V.L. and Zimmerman, S., 2008. Spiritual care at the end of life in long-term care. *Medical Care*, 46(1), pp. 85–91.

Davie, G., 2015. *Religion in Britain: A persistent paradox*. Oxford: Wiley-Blackwell.

Department of Health, 2003. *Tackling health inequalities: A programme for action*. London, UK: Department of Health.

du Boulay, S., 2007. *Cicely Saunders: The founder of the modern hospice movement*, 3rd ed., London, UK: Ashford.

Ehrenreich, J.H., 2014. *The altruistic imagination: A history of social work and social policy in the United States*. Ithaca, NY: Cornell University Press.

Engel, G.L., 1977. The need for a new medical model: A challenge for biomedicine. *Science*, 196(4286), pp. 129–136.

Eustler, N.E. and Martinez, J.M., 2003. The interdisciplinary team. In Forman, W.B., Kitzes, J.A., Anderson, R.P. and Sheehan, D.K. (eds.), *Hospice and palliative care: Concepts and practice*. Sudbury, MA: Jones and Bartlett, pp. 13–33.

Feifel, H. (ed.), 1959. *The meaning of death*. Maidenhead, UK: McGraw-Hill.

Ferrell, B., Otis-Green, S. and Economou, D., 2013. Spirituality in cancer care at the end of life. *The Cancer Journal*, 19(5), pp. 431–437.

Forman, W., Kitzes, J.A., Anderson, R.P. and Sheehan, D.K. (eds.), 2003. *Hospice and palliative care: Concepts and practice*, 2nd ed. Sudbury, MA: Jones and Bartlett.

Gordon, T. and Mitchell, D., 2004. A competency model for the assessment and delivery of spiritual care. *Palliative Medicine*, 18(7), pp. 646–651.

Gorer, G., 1955. The pornography of death. *Encounter*, 5(4), pp. 49–52.

Guyau, J.M., 2015. *The non-religion of the future: A sociological study*, vol. 39. New York, NY: Henry Holt.

Healy, L.M., 2008. Exploring the history of social work as a human rights profession. *International Social Work*, 51(6), 735–748.

Hollins, S., 2006. *Religions, culture and healthcare: A practical handbook for use in healthcare environments*. Oxon, UK: Radcliffe.

Howard, V., 2001. A holistic approach to pain. *Nursing Times*, 97(34), p. 34. Available at: http://www.nursingtimes.net/a-holistic-approach-to-pain/200675.article.

James, V. and Field, D., 1996. Who has the power? Some problems and issues affecting the nursing care of dying patients. *European Journal of Cancer Care*, 5(2), pp. 73–80.

James, N. and Field, D., 1992. The routinization of hospice: Charisma and bureaucratization. *Social Science & Medicine*, 34(12), pp. 1363–1375.

Kellehear, A., 2000. *Experiences near death: Beyond medicine and religion*. Brisbane, Australia: Replica Books.

Kennedy, P. and Kennedy, C., 2014. *Using theory to explore health, medicine and society*. Bristol, UK: Policy Press.

Kübler-Ross, E., 1969. *On death and dying*. New York, NY: Collier Books.

Lee, L., 2012. Research note: Talking about a revolution: Terminology for the new field of non-religion studies. *Journal of Contemporary Religion*, 27(1), pp. 129–139.

McPeak, C., 2003. Spiritual care of the dying person. In Forman, W.B., Kitzes, J.A., Anderson, R.P. and Sheehan, D.K. (eds.), *Hospice and palliative care: Concepts and practice*. Sudbury, MA: Jones and Bartlett, pp. 119–127.

McSherry, W., 2001. Spiritual crisis? Call a nurse. In Orchard, H. (ed.), *Spirituality in health care contexts*. London, UK: Jessica Kingsley, pp. 107–117.

McSherry, W., 1998. Nurses' perceptions of spirituality and spiritual care. *Nursing Standard*, 13(4), pp. 36–40.

McSherry, W., Cash, K. and Ross, L., 2004. Meaning of spirituality: Implications for nursing practice. *Journal of Clinical Nursing*, 13(8), pp. 934–941.

McSherry, W. and Draper, P., 1998. The debates emerging from the literature surrounding the concept of spirituality as applied to nursing. *Journal of Advanced Nursing*, 27(4), pp. 683–691.

McPeak, C., 2003. Spiritual care of the dying person. In Forman, W.B., Kitzes, J.A., Anderson, R.P. and Sheehan, D.K. (eds.), *Hospice and palliative care: Concepts and practice*. Sudbury, MA: Jones and Bartlett, pp. 119–127.

Nolan, S., 2012. *Spiritual care at the end of life: The chaplain as a 'hopeful presence'*. London, UK: Jessica Kingsley.

Paley, J., 2008. The concept of spirituality in palliative care: An alternative view. *International Journal of Palliative Nursing*, 14(9), pp. 448–452.

Parkes, C.M., 2013. Elisabeth Kübler-Ross, On death and dying: A reappraisal. *Mortality*, 18(1), pp. 94–97.

Pentaris, P., 2018. The marginalisation of religion in end of life care: Signs of microaggression? *International Journal of Human Rights in Healthcare*, 11(2), pp. 116–128.

Pentaris, P., 2014. Religion, secularism, and professional practice. *Studia Sociologica*, 6(1), pp. 99–109.

Public Health England, 2016. Faith at end of life: A resource for professionals, providers and commissioners working in community. Available at: https://www.gov.uk/government/uploads/system/uploads/attachment_data/file/496231/Faith_at_end_of_life_-_a_resource.pdf.

Puchalski, C.M., 2013. Integrating spirituality into patient care: An essential element of personcentered care. *Polskie Archiwum Medycyny Wewnetrznej*, 123(9), pp. 491–497.

Puchalski, C., Ferrell, B., Virani, R., Otis-Green, S., Baird, P., Bull, J., Chochinov, H., Handzo, G., Nelson-Becker, H., Prince-Paul, M. and Pugliese, K., 2009. Improving the quality of spiritual care as a dimension of palliative care: The report of the Consensus Conference. *Journal of Palliative Medicine*, 12(10), pp. 885–904.

Puchalski, C.M., Lunsford, B., Harris, M.H. and Miller, R.T., 2006. Interdisciplinary spiritual care for seriously ill and dying patients: A collaborative model. *The Cancer Journal*, 12(5), pp. 398–416.

Ross, L., 2006. Spiritual care in nursing: An overview of the research to date. *Journal of Clinical Nursing*, 15(7), pp. 852–862.

Saunders, D.C.M., 2006. *Cicely Saunders: Selected writings 1958–2004*. Oxford, UK: Oxford University Press.

Saunders, C., 2001. The evolution of palliative care. *Journal of the Royal Society of Medicine*, 94(9), pp. 430–432.

Saunders, C., 1996. A personal therapeutic journey. *BMJ: British Medical Journal*, 313(7072), pp. 1599–1601.

Saunders, C., 1991. *Hospice and palliative care: An interdisciplinary approach*. London, UK: Edward Arnold.

Saunders, C., 1990. *Hospice and palliative care: The principles of interdisciplinary work*. London, UK: Hodder General Publishing Division.

Saunders, C., 1988. Spiritual pain. *Journal of Palliative Care*, 4(3), pp. 29–32.

Saunders, C., 1958. Dying of cancer. *St. Thomas's Hospital Gazette*, 56(2), pp. 37–47.

Seymour, J., Clark, D. and Winslow, M., 2005. Pain and palliative care: The emergence of new specialties. *Journal of Pain and Symptom Management*, 29(1), pp. 2–13.

Simsen, B.J., 1986. The spiritual dimension. *Nursing Times*, 82(48), pp. 41–42.

Smart, N., 1996. *Dimensions of the sacred: An anatomy of the world's beliefs*. San Francisco, CA: University of California Press.

Stevenson, D.G., Huskamp, H.A., Grabowski, D.C. and Keating, N.L., (2007). Differences in hospice care between home and institutional settings. *Journal of Palliative Medicine*, 10(5), pp. 1040–1047.

Torrens, P.R., 1985. *Hospice programs and public policy*. Chicago, IL: American Hospital Publishing.

Walter, T., 2002. Spirituality in palliative care: Opportunity or burden? *Palliative Medicine*, 16(2), pp. 133–140.

Walter, T., 1999. *On bereavement: The culture of grief*. Buckingham, UK: Open University Press.

Walter, T., 1997. The ideology and organization of spiritual care: Three approaches. *Palliative Medicine*, 11(1), pp. 21–30.

White, K.L., Williams, T.F. and Greenberg, B.G., 1961. The ecology of medical care. *New England Journal of Medicine*, 265(18), pp. 885–892.

WHO Definition of Palliative Care. (2012, January 28). Retrieved from http://www.who.int/cancer/palliative/definition/en/

Wynne, L., 2013. Spiritual care at the end of life. *Nursing Standard*, 28(2), pp. 41–45.

Yardley, S.J., Walshe, C.E. and Parr, A., 2009. Improving training in spiritual care: A qualitative study exploring patient perceptions of professional educational requirements. *Palliative Medicine*, 23(7), pp. 601–607.

2 Religion and belief: A changing landscape

Introduction

This second chapter begins with the observations of many contemporary scholars that the roles and place of religion and belief in society have changed. Such changes are intense and extensive, and, therefore, 'difficult to gain a proper perspective on them' (Woodhead and Catto, 2012, p. 3). The need to acquire as much knowledge as possible – to inform practise better – is pressing, nevertheless (Fonseca and Testoni, 2011–2012). The exploration of the changing place of religion and belief is of particular importance to the progression of the arguments in this book. It prompts the conversation about how these changes have played out in professional practise, that later assists with the discussion of how religion, belief and spiritual identities are treated in EOL care nowadays.

To better understand the current place of religion and belief in society, it is imperative that a modern history of changes as delineated by several authors and researchers be explored. This discussion includes the scrutiny of two main areas: religious plurality and diversification, and the secularisation thesis. Although these narratives specify the transitions in the role of religion and belief over time, they also set the context in which religion and belief have become absent from public life (Bruce, 2011), and then present again (Davie, 2015), and finally, how our ability to talk about religion has been challenged (Dinham, 2015).

To discuss the changing landscape of religion and belief, one should find the cause first. What has led modern societies towards such complexity and multiplicity of identities and characteristics? This chapter identifies migration as the major cause of the latter and begins its exploration from there.

Migration

Meister (2011) argued that migration is the primary reason for religious diversity and plurality in developed countries. He engaged largely with interrogating the implications of the mobility of populations across nations, and concluded that two main themes emerged from that: first, the diversification of the population in the host country, and second, an undeniable need to respond to the former, but on multiple levels.

Immigration in Britain, since the 1940s, had a tremendous impact on various areas (e.g., education, welfare services, crime rates and worshiping) of the state. When World War II ended in 1945, the British economy was a priority – specifically, the recovery from losses inflicted by war (Timmins, 1995). To aid in this recovery, a large number of migrants were recruited for labour (Weller, 2007). The *Royal Commission on Population* (Redington and Clarke, 1951) reported that migrant populations can be of *good stock* and that they should be welcomed as labour. That report raised the awareness of labour market needs and, as a result, migration numbers increased.

Following the increase in the numbers, the government engaged in actions which offer a clearer picture of the changing demographics of the population – notably, the further development of the census exercise. Even though attention was given to the question associated with migration, it was still not asked in the 1951 UK Census. In the 1961 UK Census, however, a question regarding previous addresses and number of years of residency in the UK had been added (Office for National Statistics, 1977). This was due to extended demands from local authorities and the government to be conversant regarding the movement of people in the country (Office for National Statistics, 1977).

Britain welcomed migrants from several places, with the Irish community being the largest until the 1970s (for further details on other ethnicities and migration in the UK, also see Weller, 2007). But, despite their origins, people migrated to Britain for various reasons. Regardless of the motivation, the result is broadly the same or similar for every case. Immigration suggests a lot more than just a person moving from one place to another (Hansen, 2000). It encompasses a complicated adjustment, which may take time and sometimes may not even be successful. In other words, movement across nations is inclusive of the following two-sided challenge. First, migrants are challenged to acculturate to a different culture, whereas persons and communities in the host nation are challenged due to the events of enculturation – the gradual, and often unclaimed, acquisition of characteristics and traits form the migrant culture.

Both Meister (2011) and Weller (2007) acknowledged that immigration, among other things, brought increased religious plurality to the nation. Weller suggested the following:

> It was also the labour migration … that, in the 1950s and 1960s, led to workers of Hindu, Muslim and Sikh backgrounds from the Indo-Pakistani subcontinent becoming a permanent feature of UK life and bringing about the existence here of significant communities of Hindus, Muslims and Sikhs. (Weller, 2007, p. 25)

Although Weller's figures reflected the changing religious composition in the UK, his argument stressed that such movements of populations are deemed to result into nations of mixed identities and, consequentially, the need to respond to the former.

From an Anglican environment, Britain turned into a space in which the need to accommodate many and different religions was evident. The plurality raised then has been apparent to date, but with a lot more legislation and awareness in place that promotes and enhances equality within communities of multiple identities.

Religious plurality and diversification

Immigration was the cause of a series of circumstances upon which the government had to act. It is those circumstances to which we now turn – the many and various religious and nonreligious identities that gathered in a single space, without any preconceived intent to coexist. Religious plurality and diversification thus frame the context in which secular practise has thrived (Pentaris, 2014). They are the driving force of current social policy that directs service delivery in death and dying, as well as other settings.

Religious diversification grew after the 1950s, and across many nations (Davie, 2015). From a Christian plural society, the UK and Britain became religiously plural:

> It was also from the middle of the 20th century onwards that the size, distribution and significance of the other religious groups, such as Hindus, Muslims, Sikhs and Jains, grew in importance in the UK. (Weller, 2007, p. 25)

Before complete religious diversity, including minority religions, migration led a diversified number of Christian beliefs to emerge and promote Christian values and beliefs, as per the dominant. This emergence eventually resulted in the development and maintenance of a Christian plural environment.

> Thus the migration, settlement and development of new Christian communities has further diversified the profile of Christianity in England beyond even it's [*sic*] relatively (as compared with many other European countries) pluralistic Christian inheritance of *Anglican, Presbyterian, Roman Catholic* and *Free Church* traditions. (Weller, 2007, p. 23)

Apart from immigration, there are various other reasons that justify the diversity in Christian beliefs, which are still a feature of British society in the 21st century. Worth noting is the following: Christianity has undergone serious transformations that have informed and promoted the emergence of new forms of Christian life, as well as *organisational life* rooted in Christian denominations:

> As a result, the Christianity of the UK in the early twenty-first century is much more diverse than many could have imagined, even half a

century ago, both in terms of its ethnicity and the variety of its traditions, movements, denominations and other forms of organization and
presence. (Weller, 2007, p. 22)

Weller (2007) suggests that the formation of religious plurality in the UK
has taken a multifaceted course. 'Christianity in these islands has developed
into richly diverse forms' (Weller, 2007, p. 22), which later moved forward to
a state that is Christian, plural and secular all together.

Diversity within Christianity, among other religions, gained more attention in the public during the past 15 years (Woodhead and Catto, 2012). This
was magnified with the increase in visitors whose beliefs were different than
the norm. 'Individuals and groups of people belonging to other religious
traditions have come as visitors, or to live here' (Weller, 2007, p. 23). By and
large, the multiplication of religious belief in a single space became difficult
to examine. Mayo (2005, p. 16) best frames this, based on globalisation theories and the notions of migration: 'Globalization is not merely a matter
of culture and communication. Globalization is also defined in terms of
increasingly interconnected problems … which give rise to the mass movements of people'. The movement of populations, nonetheless, comes hand
in hand with the migration of social identities and personal characteristics,
but also with societal norms and beliefs that are embodied differently from
the way they were expressed in the original societies.

As discussed earlier, Britain, during the post-war period, was experiencing significantly large waves of migrants who were either seeking asylum
or migrating due to personal reasons, or were refugees (Hansen, 2000).
Migrants' unique identities and demographic characteristics, such as religion, migrated to Britain with them. The host nation faced the significant
challenge of accommodating all kinds of different religious beliefs and practises in a Christian-dominant context – a challenge that looms in contemporary public life.

Despite the success of Britain's response to this challenge, it does, today,
along with France and Germany, have the most significant decline in pro-
fessed Christian believers. Such decline is the product of the continuous
changes of the role of religion and belief in society since the post-war years.
Besides, scholars have noted that Christianity in Britain has been in crisis
since the 1960s (Meister, 2011; Erdozain, 2012; Green, 2011; Prochaska, 2006).

> In contemporary Britain Christianity may be in crisis, as many histori-
> ans and sociologists contend, but one should not assume that it is dead.
> There remains a goodly measure of belief, not least among Catholics
> and the expanding Pentecostal churches. But Christian belief is much
> less often expressed in church membership or in belonging to volun-
> tary societies. To both believers and unbelievers today, the Victorian
> assumption that competing religious institutions could stem the tide of
> social distress is baffling. (Prochaska, 2006, p. 25)

Despite the fast-paced diversification of religion and belief, the government and local authorities only started debating about the satisfaction of such needs, at a much later stage. This is primarily because all the new religions were initially distinguished by their race and ethnic diversity. Religious needs were not yet visible or alarming. The latter changed as the secondary wave of migration arrived between the 1960s and 1980s. Those migrants were the families (spouses and children) of those from the first wave. The demographic changes, the increase in the number of people from certain religious movements or creeds, led to the unavoidable need to accommodate individual desires associated with religious practises.

> This phase of migration laid the basis for the development of a range of social, cultural and religious communities and institutions that would maintain and transmit their religious traditions. Mandirs, gurdwaras and mosques were founded and became an increasingly established part of community life. (Weller, 2007, p. 25)

The identity shifts in the population highlight an enormous complexity of conscious notions within the individuals, families, smaller groups and societies. In other words, religious plurality and diversification play a key role in two areas: first, how members of an identified society perceive themselves, and in relation to others in the same environment; and second, how societies develop or maintain their resources to meet fully the needs of their subjects, such as providing suitable support in EOL care, as is this book's central point.

Religious composition today

The previous section partially highlights the premise in which the original hypothesis of this project is formulated. Religious plurality and diversification induce complex needs across several areas in society, which need adequate and proper examination. Nevertheless, it would be uncanny to approach the situation without first looking at the most recent information of the religious composition, which reflects plurality and diversity, to form a better understanding of the complexities in question.

Britain is one of the most religiously diverse countries in the European Union. It is the composition of multi-faith societies in which people have the freedom to choose their religious or nonreligious beliefs. Although Christianity remains the predominant religion in the country, other religions started taking significant hold too, such as Judaism, Hinduism, Sikhism and Islam. Table 2.1 details data from the 2011 UK Census: religious affiliation in the UK. Christianity, Islam and No Religion are the three groups that changed the most since the previous census. Christianity remains the largest religious group, with Islam following at 4.8%, whereas the number of people who state no affiliation to any religion has increased significantly to 25.1%.

Table 2.1 2011 Census: Religious affiliation in the UK

Religion/No religion	Percentage
Christian	59.3
Buddhist	0.4
Hindu	1.5
Jewish	0.5
Muslim (Islam)	4.8
Sikh	0.8
Other: Pagan	0.1
Other: Spiritualist	0.1
No religion	25.1
Agnostic	0.1
Atheist	0.1
Jedi knight	0.3
Religion not stated	7.2

Source: Office for National Statistics, UK Census 2011, n.d. Available at: http://www.ons.gov.uk/ons/datasets-and-tables/index.html?pageSize=50&sortBy=none&sortDirection=none&newquery=religion&content-type=Reference+table&content-type=Dataset.

It is, though, important to highlight that the question about religion and belief in the census is voluntary, and, therefore, we are unsure how broadly the information can be generalised. In addition, this information may change radically by the next census exercise.

The situation in the UK is not dissimilar to many other countries. For example, the *Religious Landscape Study* by the PEW Forum (PEW Research, 2012), in the US, shows that over 70% of the population report affiliation with Christianity, approximately 6% affiliate with other than Christianity religions, and people with no stated affiliation represent 22.8% of the respondents of the study.

Drawing on the earlier remark that the question about religion or belief is voluntary in the census, perhaps it is worth looking at the British Social Attitudes (BSA) about religious affiliations in Britain, along with the UK Census 2011 data. This will benefit our understanding of how people generally view religion and faith, beyond the notion of belonging.

From the information shown in Table 2.2, it is evident that even though public responses vary, two dominant categories emerge from the survey: Christianity and No Religion. Approximately 85% of the respondents chose either Christianity or No Religion. The division between the two is almost equal, with approximately 3,200 people stating affiliation with Christianity or no affiliation at all. The number of people who state they do not affiliate with any religion is increasing, and, based on the BSA survey, is larger than what the UK census depicts.

Despite the claim that Britain is a Christian country, a notion discussed earlier in this chapter, the 31st annual BSA survey (conducted in 2014) found

Table 2.2 British Social Attitudes Survey 2013: Do you regard yourself as belonging to any particular religion? Which?

Response	Number
No religion	1,558
Christian – no denomination	381
Roman Catholic	288
Church of England/Anglican	636
Baptist	15
Methodist	48
Presbyterian/Church of Scotland	66
Other Christian	7
Hindu	32
Jewish	16
Muslim	106
Sikh	7
Buddhist	13
Other non-Christian	14
Free Presbyterian	1
Other Protestant	36
Don't know	2

Source: UK Data Service, n.d. British Social Attitudes Survey, 2013. Available at: https://discover.ukdataservice.ac.uk/variables/?q=%22do% 20you%20regard%20yourself%20as%20belonging%20to%20any% 20particular%20religion%22%20SeriesTitle:British%20Social% 20Attitudes%20Survey#7809_V392 (retrieved 26 February 2017).

that over 50% of the population state they have no religion, as opposed to 41.7% who claim affiliation with Christianity.

It is apparent that there are discrepancies between social attitudes and the data from the census. This may be due to how attitudes are influenced by how we understand religious affiliation and belonging, or the number of respondents for each survey. Regardless of the reason, the high numbers of people who state they either belong or not to a religion or denomination is part of the service user population seeking assistance and support in death and dying settings, as well as the EOL experts who provide the services. This heightens the importance of addressing the challenges that healthcare professionals (HCP) face when it is necessary to engage with religion, belief and spiritual identities of service users. In other words, the process of familiarising with the complexity and religious composition of a population is a resource for action. It provides knowledge which might influence decision-making in policy and practise. It is one of these areas we turn to next: changing demographics of experts in hospice care.

Religious diversity and hospice care

Migration not only affected religious life and the composition of the nation, but also it impacted on the diversification of hospice professionals.

Individual migrants arrived in the UK with either specialist knowledge in end of life care, which was later recognised by the respective regulatory bodies in the UK (e.g., Health and Care Professions Council [HCPC]), or the intention to train in this area of practise, whether medical or non-medical training, and later apply their knowledge in the field.

According to the statistics from The Migration Observatory (2015), the overall share of first-generation migrants in total employment increased over the years to 16.7%, in 2015, with the projection to increase more. Of this number, 26% (1.7% occupation share) are health professionals, including physicians and nurses, as well as allied professionals. However, the information from the Observatory does not provide explicit data about migrants' religious or faith backgrounds, which makes it difficult to estimate the diversification in this area.

Data from the 2001 Census (Office for National Statistics, UK Census 2011, n.d.) show that healthcare personnel were mostly of White ethnicity (70% of doctors, 81% of dentists, 89% of nurses, 89% of midwives and 90% of other staff in the healthcare sector) – whether British White or Other White is not confirmed, however. On the other side, only 10% of staff in the healthcare sector identified as Non-white, exclusive of 30% of doctors and 11% of nurses. Of course, these statistics only offer an idea of ethnic background, but due to scarce data regarding religion, it is uncertain what the religious or belief characteristics of healthcare professionals are.

Having said that, the Office for National Statistics, UK Census 2011 (n.d.) drew from the Census 2011 data and presented workforce by religion. The information in Table 2.3 concerns the whole of England, whereas Table 2.4 refers to London, where the study informing this book took place.

Without doubt, these statistics, once again, are not representative of the workforce in EOL care, inclusive of hospices, palliative care units in hospitals, care homes and community services. Nevertheless, it is with confidence that we can assume the following. Non-white personnel in the healthcare sector, whose ethnic background is other than British, are more

Table 2.3 Workforce in England by religion (Census 2011)

Religion	Workforce (in numbers)
Christian	14,694,608
Buddhist	126,747
Hindu	421,985
Jewish	118,617
Muslim	811,749
Sikh	209,632
Other religion	127,480
No religion	6,872,882
Not stated	1,704,143

Source: Office for National Statistics, n.d. Available at http://www. nomisweb.co.uk/census/2011/WP210EW/view/2092957699?cols=measures.

Table 2.4 Workforce in London by religion (Census 2011)

Religion	Workforce (in numbers)
Christian	2,264,756
Buddhist	44,276
Hindu	211,848
Jewish	72,015
Muslim	309,824
Sikh	65,946
Other religion	28,711
No religion	1,149,234
Not stated	353,871

Source: Office for National Statistics, n.d. Available at http://www.nomisweb. co.uk/census/2011/WP210EW/view/2013265927?cols=measures.

likely to identify with other than Christian religions. Equally, though, many healthcare practitioners with a White ethnicity may identify with a different-than-Christianity religion – most notably, no religion.

Last, it is worth noting that hospice professionals will be a much smaller number of the healthcare staff statistics indicated in these tables. Their practise varies based on the place in which people die (Gomes and Higginson, 2008), something that is discussed extensively later in this book. For the benefit of the current discussion, however, I should highlight that there is a dearth of information about professionals by EOL care setting (e.g., care home, hospice) and by religion. Therefore, we can only rely on the workforce statistics in Tables 2.3 and 2.4, which emphasise the diversity of identities in employment.

Concluding note

Considering the decline in religious affiliation, historians and sociologists are examining the future trends of religious connections and belonging. The estimates show that Muslims are a broad category of migrants which continually grows. This indicates a significant increase in Islam affiliations in the future (Norris, 2011; Meister, 2011). Even though Christianity, and especially Anglicanism, reflects the main religious practise in Britain, other so-called 'minority' religions co-exist and intersect with the dominant one. The most common minority religions in Britain are Judaism, Sikhism, Islam, Hinduism and Buddhism (for a more sociological discussion see Woodhead and Catto, 2012).

This chapter highlights that religious diversification is the result of migration. A religion does not just transfer to a different nation through the migration of its believers. It adapts to the societal, political and environmental circumstances of the host nation. 'Religions change as they travel, and so do those who live by them' (Woodhead and Catto, 2012, p. 86). Furthermore,

the dominant religion of the location to which one migrates is also changing and adapting to the new religious affiliations in its environment and
to the impact the new religions have. This entails a whole process of inter-
and intra-communication among faith groups and belief systems to use the
opportunity for increased knowledge and understanding of religion and
belief within a multi-faith society. If we view secularisation as a reaction
to those changes and the overall complexity of the religious composition in
Britain, then we can speculate that religion has become privatised due to
feelings of inclusion and respect to diversity (see Prothero and Kerby, 2015).
Moving forward, and addressing this speculation, which further presents
the changes religion and belief have undergone, it is important that we consider the case of religious decline more thoroughly and include secularisation and desecularisation in the conversation.

Religious decline, secularisation and desecularisation

Sociology has long reflected a widespread assumption of religious decline
(Fischoff, 1993; Luckmann, 1990; Fallding, 1974; Berger, 1967; Wilson,
1966), though the opposite has also been posited since at least the 1970s
(Martin, 1978) and continuously ever since (Davie, 1994, 2007; Berger, 1999;
Habermas and Seidman, 1989; Hervieu-Léger, 2000; Voas and Day, 2007;
Dinham, 2009; Woodhead and Catto, 2012, Dinham, 2012; Dinham and
Francis, 2015).

Wilson (1966) suggests that the social significance of religion in the public
domain has suffered in modernity and was eventually lost. In these terms,
secularisation is a process of religious decline in public life, which in turn
is an unavoidable consequence of modernity. Similarly, Berger (1967) identified that despite religion's importance in providing a unifying belief and
worldview, the process of secularisation has had a conflicting impact on
individuals and society. Berger (1967, p. 107) defined secularisation as 'the
process by which sectors of society and culture are removed from the dom-
ination of religious institutions and symbols', whereas later he termed the
freedom to choose affiliation to a religious denomination the 'heretical
imperative' (Berger and Luckmann, 1981).

Fallding (1974) identifies 'inclusive' and 'exclusive' religion. The former is
closer to the shapes of new religions and new spiritualities – a more individualised experience of belief. On the other hand, exclusive religion indicates
decline, also as described earlier. In addition, Fischoff (1993) and Luckmann
(1990) both suggest religious decline. Luckmann (1990) also recognises the
changes that modernity brought to the social construction of society and,
therefore, suggests that religion is no longer the centre of attention due to
these structural changes.

Martin (1978), however, argues that secularisation has served a primarily
ideological purpose, with limited proof of religious decline. This argument
has caused further debate and ambiguity in the field. Beyond this point,

Davie (1994, p. 2) introduces her thesis on believing without belonging, arguing that 'the majority of British people – in common with many other Europeans – persist in believing (if only in an ordinary God), but see no need to participate with even minimal regularity in their religious institutions'. This may be complementary to the reasons why people state no religious affiliation in the census. Whether affiliation is linked with practise, and not belief, is a question that Day (2010) attempted to answer some 15 years later.

In contrast, Voas and Day (2007) identify religious changes as the corruption of religions in their proper form, into a fuzzy form which they term 'fuzzy fidelity' (also see Voas, 2009). Over 10 years after her *believing without belonging* thesis, Davie (2007, p. 22) moves beyond it, suggesting vicarious religion which she defines as 'the notion of religion performed by an active minority but on behalf of a much larger number, who (implicitly at least) not only understand, but, quite clearly, approve of what the minority is doing'. In other words, vicarious religion concerns religious practise by churches and church leaders on behalf of others. Examples of this include a marriage, a funeral, or a christening, all of which require a form of consent by the vast majority.

In a different approach, Rowan Williams' (2006) observations include 'programmatic' versus 'procedural' secularisation. Programmatic secularism refers to a deliberate, conscious decision to be secular: 'when the Church is regarded as an enemy ... that must be resolutely excluded from public debate, liberal modernity turns itself into a fixed and absolute thing, another pseudo-religion' (Williams, 2006, p. 79). On the other hand, procedural secularism is behaving on the assumption that things are secular. In both cases, secularism persists, and intensifies the changes religion and belief have undergone to date.

Some 30 years after his first argument on the social reality of religion (Berger, 1967), Berger (1999) suggested that his analyses were misled by his own thinking. He suggested that society is as religious as ever. He did this by introducing the desecularisation thesis. Others (Hervieu-Léger, 2000; Woodhead and Catto, 2012; Davie, 2013; Day, 2010; Dinham, 2009; Martin, 2005), in various and different ways, but also for various reasons, suggested that religion never went away, but rather has changed.

Secularisation theories have suggested that whilst societies advance they will become more secular (Beyer, 1994). On the same note, several commentators of sociology have noted that religion may be in a permanent decline. The founders of sociology, Karl Marx (1818–1883), Èmile Durkheim (1857–1917) and Max Weber (1864–1920), have all noted this process of religious decline. However, the examination of religious decline and modernisation has been undertaken by, and for, a Christian-dominated world. These two terms – 'religion' and 'Christianity' – have the tendency to be linked in conversations and even used interchangeably. Bruce (2002) argues about secular beliefs based on western and Christian-oriented communities, for example. However, commentary on minority religions is limited.

Despite its recent evidence, secularisation has already found its counter-process. Berger (1999) has discussed his thesis of how secular beliefs and privatised patterns of religious behaviours are turning around again as people adopt more *desecular* beliefs. As noted by Karpov (2010), Berger's thesis was expected to initiate an emergence of research questions and hypotheses, and it did. It is worth noting here, though, that desecularisation-related research and theoretical approach rapidly became relevant to the sociology of religion but has not been used as much by research on public professions.

Berger (1999) describes the concept of desecularisation as 'counter-secularisation' and has 'offered an innovative view of the vitality of religion vis-à-vis global modernity' (Karpov, 2010; p. 232). Desecularisation implies that the secular assumptions have been wrong and that communities, as they modernise, remain as religious as ever (Berger, 1999).

With desecularisation theories, predictions of inexorable secularisation have been undermined (Woodhead and Catto, 2012). Karpov debates the latter suggestion by exploring the definition of Berger's desecularisation thesis:

> Theorizing desecularization does not involve an all-out refutation of the secularization thesis ... a valid conceptualization of desecularization as counter-secularization rests upon acknowledging the presence of secularization trends and forces. Only in such a manner will we be able to approach the important task of studying the interplay between secularizing and counter-secularizing trends. Therefore, the development of a theory of desecularization will ... benefit once this issue is detached more clearly from the never-ending debate on whether or not and to what extent secularization is a reality. (Karpov, 2010, p. 237)

Desecularisation, in other words, is a process of reacknowledgement of the social significance of religion and belief, in the public sphere; it is the recognition that secularism is no longer pertinent to 21st-century societies, and that religion and belief are in the core of individual and public life.

Further beyond the discussion about the secular, Habermas (2008) argues that societies are now post-secular – in other words, concerned with the relationship between religious and secular beliefs. Beaumont and Baker (2011, p. 2) present the post-secular city as a space where the role and boundaries of religion are 'no longer rigidly enforced .... and new relations of possibility are emerging'. Preceding this claim is Beaumont's suggestion that the post-secular

> does not infer that we now live in a radically different age compared with half a century ago ... the limits of the secularization thesis and the ever-growing realization of radically plural societies in terms of religion, faith and belief within and between diverse urban societies. If we consider postsecular as the indication of diverse religious, humanist and secularist positionalities ... it is precisely the relations between

these dimensions and not just the religious that are taken into account. (Beaumont, 2010, p. 6)

On the other hand, Beckford describes Habermas' claims as paternalistic:

Habermas insists that religious contributions to public debate must be translatable into the supposedly neutral language of secular reason. He wants to exclude direct or untranslated religious voices from legislatures, courts of law and public bureaucracies. He accepts that public religions are enjoying a resurgence but he would also like to prevent them from exercising power where it really matters. This represents an emasculation of the public sphere. (Beckford, 2010, p. 125)

In other words, according to Beckford (2010), Habermas describes the post-secular as a state in which religious contribution is communicated with neutral terms. I will share Beckford's scepticism here, for neutral terminology and avoidance of religious character appear to facilitate religious illiteracy in different parts of public society, rather than being inclusive, acknowledging and engaging with diversity, as is the consensus of this volume.

As societies modernise and develop, they view religion, along with race, ethnicity and other matters, in a different way. As social coherence evolves and multi-culturalism has settled in today's communities, religion is treated in the way expected to meet the needs of the new social structures and social functioning. According to Stackhouse (2011, p. 239), 'religions have been moderated or otherwise manipulated by modern powers in various respects to suit various agendas'. In these terms, secularisation, desecularisation and the post-secular may refer to a societal needs assessment and the necessity of adjusting religious beliefs and values to current public desires. Secularisation may as well refer to the desire for better adjustment to societal changes, as opposed to an informed individualistic decision to privatise religion. Of course, these are claims yet to be explored.

Green (2011), based on his historical and more empirical evidence of religious change in the modernised religious world, argues that the process of secularisation commenced with the elimination of religious questions within politics. The expulsion of these questions has had an important impact on the modern social history of religion. In support of my previous assumptions and also Stackhouse's work (2011), the privatisation of religion and the adoption of secular beliefs may be the product of the new challenges emerging in the multi-faith communities and multi-cultural contexts that shape modern societies.

The lack of causation of the secularisation paradigm is heavily critiqued by Bruce (2011), who *complains* that he has presented enough statistical evidence to answer the question *why*. However, others do not share this view (Green, 2011; Erdozain, 2012; Warner, Van Antwerpen and Calhoun, 2010). To illustrate theoretically a concept of the secularisation causality, it is necessary to combine a few different ideas (Erdozain, 2012) and find the interconnections with the trends in secular beliefs. The following sections present the most important concepts for helping us understand the interconnections and the effect these processes have had on the causality of secularisation, in relation to EOL care, and hospice care specifically.

Nonreligion

Another field of study which emerged in the discussion about religious decline regards nonreligion, even though the ongoing dialogue in this area uses terms interchangeably (e.g., secular, atheism, irreligion, nonreligion). The exploration of nonreligion is not new, but only recently has it been revisited systematically in literature, which makes it important to discuss here.

Guyau (2015) described religion as a form of social relation, an extension of human life, highlighting the relationships between men and gods. He defined religion as follows:

> [It] is an imaginative extension, a universalization of all the good and evil relations which exist among conscious beings, of war and peace, friendship and enmity, obedience and rebellion, protection and authority, submission, fear, respect, devotion, love: religion is a universal *sociomorphism*. (Guyau, 2015, p. 2)

There is indeed much truth in this definition, but it also tends to apply more with polytheism and not monotheism – a binary most prominent in discussions about nonreligion.

Guyau (2015) opined that religion was no longer important, since the 19th century, and it was only a matter of time before societies disregard it. In his explorations of religion, Guyau focussed on why religion is facing the ultimate extinction in the world, based on its social and functional roles, and argued that this extinction signified the emergence of a new concept: nonreligion.

Nonreligion is a fast-growing field of research and scientific study, yet remains dubious to many as it does not always conform to the conventional ideas presented in the sociology of religion or related fields. Similar to Guyau's non-conventional thoughts, Campbell (1971) argued that irreligion was allied to the nonreligion field, emphasising the active rejection of traditions that are religious. Campbell's work is radical in the sense that it comes to contest the public's engagement or disengagement with religion, but suggests the public opposes themselves to religion. In other words, in the literature of nonreligion, irreligion is a concept dependent on the presence, and not absence, of religion. Similarly, Quack (2014), more recently, proposed a programmatic approach to the study of nonreligion which purportedly referred to what Campbell identified as irreligion. Quack's approach suggests that nonreligion can be studied based on its relationship with religiosity. He recommends that one's nonreligiousness can only be measured in relation to a person's way of connecting to religion.

Popular in the sociology of religion literature is that nonreligion refers to the absence of religious belief or religious tradition. Bullivant and Lee (2012) highlighted the emerging field of nonreligion rather recently and how it separates from secular concepts. They argued that nonreligion is not an equivalent to secularism or secularity. They distinguish these into sub-fields and recommend that better care needs be taken in literature. Lee (2012), besides putting further emphasis on the rapid evolvement of the field of nonreligion, drew attention to the limited definitional development. She argues that the term 'nonreligion' is used 'inconsistently, imprecisely, and often illogically' (Lee, 2012, abstract). She opines that this a confusing approach that does little justice to the scientific explorations of nonreligion and recommends the use of the term 'nonreligion' as an umbrella of the field, inclusive of the study of secularism, secularity and atheism.

Recently, Jong (2015) offered a conceptual dialogue about the definition or not of religion or nonreligion, as well as all related terms (e.g., secular, secularism, atheism). Jong argues that religion and all the social phenomena associated with it are fuzzy concepts, difficult to define; hence, scholars should abstain from attempting such definitions and accept the uniquely described nature of all such terms.

Secularisation and professional practise

As we go through the causality of secularisation, it is important that links be made with the secular context of professional practise. The context wherein the expertise of professional practitioners is built reflects secular characteristics, practises designed for service users under the assumption that individuals have become less and less religious, and do not, to a great extent, interpret their life experiences (e.g., death) through the lens of their faith. Looking at the concepts that boosted the secularisation process will enhance our understanding of the current position of religious or nonreligious matters within hospice care.

Some critiques of religious decline recognise that religion has remained fully present in society, though changing continuously in its role and effect, and that, concomitantly, people have largely lost their ability to engage with it. Dinham (2015) articulates this as lack of religious literacy, highlighting its impact on an inability to produce appropriate language and policies that respond to the needs of religiously plural and diversified societies. Lack of understanding of the role of religion and belief may lead to limited skills and abilities to engage with it, and result in poor quality of services and service delivery. The remainder of this section provides an exhaustive account of the concept religious literacy and highlights its use in the exploration of the place of religion in hospice care.

Religious literacy

Dinham and Francis (2015, p. 257) describe religious literacy as 'a fluid notion' that can be understood in the context in which it happens, as well as a concept that 'requires a willingness to recognise it as relevant' (Dinham and Francis, 2015, p. 11). This poses two great challenges. How do we go about quantifying religious literacy? If *fluidity* describes religious literacy, then this is a concept that is probably not easily examined in policy or practise terms – two areas in which unambiguous and explicit information and guidelines are necessary. Furthermore, the recognition of religious literacy should appear in a tangible, more concrete form so it can be comprehended more widely. Both these challenges are examined whilst this volume progresses from the first part to the next. With this in mind, it is only appropriate to provide a discussion about the different conceptions of religious literacy, which reflect religious change as discussed earlier in this chapter.

Prothero and Kerby (2015) place religious literacy in the loss of religious tradition but not religion itself. They delve into the history of protestant Americans and interrogate the absence of engagement with religious traditions in public life, with distinguishing examples from politics and school life. These examples are used to illustrate the point that 'the devotion of Americans to tolerance and inclusiveness have caused them to forget much of what they once knew about their own religious tradition' (Prothero and Kerby, 2015, p. 57). However, 'religious literacy does not have to come at the price of religious harmony' (Prothero and Kerby, 2015, p. 64). Their argument is compatible with the idea that people should re-engage with their traditions, and thus become more religious literate, and explore the possibility of developing a more tolerant attitude towards minority religious groups; 'religious literacy can also lead to a more robust tolerance, particularly for minority religious groups who do not fit into the Protestant model that has dominated American religious history' (Prothero and Kerby, 2015, p. 74).

According to Moore (2015, p. 27), 'an important dimension of diminishing religious illiteracy is to provide resources for *how to recognise, understand, and analyse* religious influences in contemporary life'. This is better understood if we look at her earlier definition of religious literacy. Moore's interpretation is that religious literacy explores the intersected areas of religion, culture, political and social life (Moore, 2006). In other words, levels of religious literacy cannot increase unless explored from the perspective that it is embedded and influences each aspect of life – primarily, culture. It is fundamental that religions and religious influences are understood 'in context and as inextricably woven into all dimensions of human experience' (Moore, 2015, p. 31).

Another conception is offered by Dinham (2015) in his account regarding religion and welfare. Dinham uses the welfare lens to present the enigma of religious literacy in public life:

> This is the conundrum of religious literacy as it presents through the welfare lens. It confronts the public sphere with the urgent need to re-skill its public professionals and citizens for the daily encounter with the full range of religious plurality. (Dinham, 2015, p. 110)

Dinham's argument is rooted in the post-war years, and notably during the fertilisation of the welfare state. The division between the state and the Church, as well as the differentiation of their roles have led to a newly formed context in which professionals are trained without the knowledge of the interplay of religion and belief in their practise. Dinham concludes that due to limited or no attention to religion and belief for a long period, professionals have lost their ability to talk about religion, and now find it hard to re-engage. Religious literacy for Dinham (2015) is the engagement with a complex society, both secular and religious, and it starts with recognising the importance and relevance of this to public life.

On the other hand, Ford and Higton (2015) explore theology and religious studies as tools that can be used in the journey towards religious literacy. They do not in any way suggest that these two areas depict religious literacy, but add value to the conversation about religion. They conclude that religious literacy

> involves learning patterns of fruitful interaction – engaged, conversational, perhaps argumentative. It involves learning how religious communities argue, and how to join in with those arguments in order to explore agreements and disagreements, and the dynamics by which they can change. It involves engagement with questions raised about, between, by and with the religions. (Ford and Higton, 2015, p. 52)

Religious literacy is a notion that is contested, and its contestations stem from the arguments that followed the theories of secularisation, as well as from the thesis that religion has lost significance. This presumption – the lost significance of religion – resulted in the classical secularisation theory (Wilson, 1966; also see Taylor, 2007) and prolonged discussions about religious decline and disengagement from the public. The consequences were many in public life, including lack of engagement with religion and belief (Dinham and Francis, 2015). Public professions have gradually lost literacy – the appropriate language to address religion and belief, whether in policy or practise. However, religion and belief continue to impact on individual consciousness and public life (Davie, 2015). The largest part of the population – worldwide, 84% – reports religious affiliation (PEW Research, 2012). On a parallel note, a readdressing of religion and belief in the public sphere is evident since the late 1990s (Berger, 1999), but with tremendous challenges. At a time when people considered religion and belief important aspects of life, they are also faced with their lost ability to talk about it. Dinham (2015, p. 108) coins this as 'anxious re-visibility'.

In underpinning religious literacy, it is also important to highlight the areas in which religion and belief have been misunderstood to be absent from public life recently. Often, people might be religious and believe, but not by practising or being affiliated with either religious establishments or religious activities (Davie, 1994). As secularisation theories suggest, this is a case of private religious matters (Martin, 1978). The census data only depicts the answers of (1) people who decided to answer, as the question of religious affiliation is not mandatory; and (2) people who affiliate, or not, themselves with a religious establishment, or activity, social action or sense of belonging.

Even though people do not affiliate with religions as much as they did before (Office for National Statistics, UK Census 2011), the subject of religion is often included in public discourse (Dinham, 2009). There is a universal lack of understanding of religion, however; its presence and interconnections with different walks of life (Garces-Foley, 2006). At a time when religious diversity has increased (Weller, 2007; Meister, 2011) and as society becomes more complicated as it modernises, and although secularity (Wilson, 1966; Bruce, 2011), desecularisation (Berger, 1999) and the post-secular (Beaumont and Baker, 2011) coincide in the discourse, religious literacy has become more important than ever.

> Religious literacy is a pressing need across society, in the full range of sectors and settings. Religion and belief, the private and the public, religion and the secular, are not separate but inescapably bound up – in law, in identities, in beliefs and in practices, not to mention the physical landscape, with its spires, mosques and temples. (Dinham and Francis, 2015, p. 11)

Worth noting is the following. People who claimed no religious affiliation constitute another unique category that should not be ignored in religious literacy discourses. Lack of affiliation with a religion may as well refer to spiritual meaning-making through the life course (Canda and Furman, 2010), as opposed to following the readings of a creed. In spite of people's affiliation or lack thereof, secular ideas and beliefs increase ambivalence towards religion. 'Resistance by secular partners to consultation with, and the incorporation of, faith groups in the policy frame may reflect ongoing mistrust as well as lack of religious literacy' (Baker, 2009, p. 108). According to Berger (1999, p. 11), 'religion is the human enterprise by which a sacred cosmos is established' and by which people make meaning and sense of their communal, social, political and personal relationships and experiences.

According to Dinham and Francis (2015, p. 11), 'it is impossible to talk fully about the public sphere without talking about religion and belief'. Religious literacy requires, as the first step, recognition that 'religion and belief pervade as majority, normal and mainstream, whatever one's own position or stance' (Dinham and Francis, 2015, p. 11). Drawing from Beyer's (1994) typology of religion, the latter may be a societal or a cultural system. People do not cope well with religion when it is treated as culture. In the space of professional practise, there are different theories and models when responding to cultural versus religious traditions and beliefs. Nonetheless, both are relevant to public professions that engage with service user identities, such is hospice care.

Moore (2015, p. 29) suggests that 'religions are collections of ideas, practises, values and stories that are all embedded in cultures and not separable from them'. However, religion as a culture retains customs and rituals in one's life despite the personal preference of non-affiliation. For example, people still get married or celebrate Vesak (Buddha Day). These are all traditional forms of practise that represent religious doctrines, nevertheless not treated as such necessarily.

The contested notion of religious literacy may also be approached differently at different times and places in which it is contextually relevant. Some interesting accounts include Prothero and Kerby (2015), as explored earlier. They consider religious literacy to be the loss of knowledge about traditions, first located in Christianity. They suggest that religious literacy intends to increase tolerance in society. Similarly, hospice care involves approaches that find solutions to the challenging multi-faith service user population. Knowledge about religions will not result in religious literacy. Contrary to Prothero and Kerby (2015), loss of knowledge about traditions in hospice care did not lead to religious illiteracy, but rather facilitated the tendency to avoid the subject further, as we see in later chapters.

Different from Prothero's and Kerby's (2015) conception, Barnes and Smith (2015, p. 85) approach religious literacy as harmony: 'acquiring religious literacy requires a positive and relational encounter with people from different faiths and beliefs'. They suggest that diversity among people should not be suppressed, nor omitted. Public life should value difference and embrace the possibilities that will lead towards harmony. This is relevant to the thesis of this volume for it supports the argument that religious diversification in hospice care should be valued with acknowledgement and facilitation towards harmonious existence and understanding.

The modern history of the welfare state shows that religious language gradually disappeared from care, and a secular-minded dialogue took its place (Dinham, 2015). 'Public professionals such as the new NHS doctors, social workers and state-employed teachers had taken on the care functions of the churches' (Dinham, 2015, p. 106). This supports the argument that professionals who practise in death and dying settings have received a secular-minded education that has left them precarious of properly engaging with religion, belief and spiritual identities of service users. This statement is further scrutinised in the subsequent chapters.

Implications of religious plurality

Woodhead and Catto (2012, p. 86) suggest, as pointed out earlier in the text, that 'when religions move, it is not merely a case of transporting a fixed body of beliefs and practises unchanged from a place of origin to a new location'.

That said, religious plurality increased over the decades and caused irritation and conflict within the community (Wohlrab-Sahr, 2003). 'The more this happens, the more important is the question of how we look at diversity, how we evaluate it and deal with it' (Portmann and Plüss, 2011, pp. 180–181). The emergence of multiple religions in the nation caused an intense situation of acculturation of religion and belief. The government, however, did not account, at the time, for the implications that such a religious movement would have.

> Community is a fundamental dimension of spirituality and religion, not only as a beneficial factor for the individual engaging the world, but also while offering an alternative perspective or rather a different 'focus' on ways of engaging life. Groups of people sharing common values, sharing interest in particular spiritualities or sharing different worldviews and acting together toward a common goal, truly impacts their members. (Champagne, 2009, p. 1)

According to Weller (2007), the core focus of social policy, upon the immigration waves and plural identities, was race and ethnicity, but not religion. More and more faith groups were included in society (Weller, 2007), and engagement in social action was cherished (Dinham, 2012). However, such religious diversity brought up matters of adjustment in sectors such as health and social care, political, and so on – things that were not necessarily explored in the Beveridge Report (BR) as it was thought through in the postwar period (see Timmins, 1995).

The End of Life Care Strategy 2008 is a good example to show how the government identified the need for addressing the unique experiences of death, dying and bereavement (DDB) in relation to individual identities and how these were taken into a considerate plan of social policy. This strategy suggests that individuals adapt their attitudes towards death, the process of dying and bereavement adjustments. These attitudes may be driven by multiple different factors: religion, culture, ethnicity, past experiences and many more. The Index for Personal Preferences recognises these and integrates new dimensions in EOL care (NHS England, 2014), inclusive of hospice care.

The Equality Act 2010 incorporated religion and belief as valuable factors of social justice and equality. The Equality and Human Rights Commission is now working on multiple projects, which relate to religious and spiritual beliefs intersected with various aspects of life. A good example of such projects is the Muslim Women Power List. The List, inaugurated in 2009, celebrated the growing number of Muslim employed women in the UK at the time; it exceeded 100,000. Another example is the New Guidance on Religion or Belief (ECHR, 2013), which was released in February 2013 by the European Court of Human Rights, to be followed by the Human Rights Commissions including the Equality and Human Rights Commission (EHRC). The guidance document is based on four case studies from a Christian background, but its applicability goes across all religions and faiths.

Religious plurality has caused not only conflict and irritation within the community, but also has affected social cohesion (Cantle, 2008) and has had an impact on everyday practise (Weller, 2007). Within the same context, Britain learned to comply with the dominant religion – Christianity – and Christian faith influenced social cohesion in numerous ways (Prochaska, 2006; Green, 2011).

The recognition of religious plurality and awareness of personal identities has had broad implications (Woodhead and Catto, 2012) and reflects the need to re-assess professional practise and its course within the experiences of DDB. Religious literacy of healthcare professionals in death and dying settings does not suggest a withdrawal of secular identities, if supported. On the contrary, it implies an increase in the awareness of religious and nonreligious individual aspects on DDB, as well as being appropriate to the challenges and shifting needs and approaches in hospice care.

References

Baker, C., 2009. Blurred encounters? Religious literacy, spiritual capital and language. In Dinham, A., Furbey, R. and Lowndes, V. (eds.), *Faith in the public realm: Controversies, policies and practices*. Bristol, UK: Policy Press, pp. 105–122.

Barnes, M. and Smith, J.D., 2015. Religious literacy as lokahi: Social harmony through diversity. In Dinham, A. and Francis, M. (eds.), *Religious literacy in policy and practice*. Bristol, UK: Policy Press, pp. 77–98.

Beaumont, J.R., 2010. Transcending the particular in postsecular cities. In Molendijk, A.L., Beaumont, J. and Jedan, C. (eds.), *Exploring the postsecular: The religious, the political and the urban*. Leiden, The Netherlands: Brill, pp. 3–17.

Beaumont, J. and Baker, C. (eds.), 2011. *Postsecular cities: Space, theory and practice*. London, UK: Continuum.

Beckford, J.A., 2010. The uses of religion in public institutions: The case of prisons. In Molendijk, A.L., Beaumont, J. and Jedan, C. (eds.), *Exploring the postsecular: The religious, the political and the urban*. Leiden, The Netherlands: Brill, pp. 383–401.

Berger, P.L., 1999. The desecularization of the world: A global overview. In Berger, P.L. (ed.), *The desecularization of the world: Resurgent religion and world politics*. Washington, DC: William B. Eerdmans, pp. 1–18.

Berger, P.L., 1967. *The social reality of religion*. London, UK: Penguin Books.

Berger, P.L. and Luckmann, T., 1981. The heretical imperative: Contemporary possibilities of religious affirmation. *Religious Studies*, 17(1), pp. 109–120.

Beyer, P., 1994. *Religion and globalization*. London, UK: SAGE.

Bruce, S., 2011. *Secularization*. New York, NY: Oxford University Press.

Bruce, S., 2002. *God is dead: Secularization in the West*. Oxford, UK: Blackwell.

Bullivant, S. and Lee, L., 2012. Interdisciplinary studies of nonreligion and secularity: The state of the union. *Journal of Contemporary Religion*, 27(1), pp. 19–27.

Campbell, C.D., 1971. *Toward a sociology of irreligion*. London: Macmillan.

Canda, E.R. and Furman, L.D., 2010. *Spiritual diversity in social work practice: The heart of helping*, 2nd ed. New York, NY: Oxford University Press.

Cantle, T., 2008. *Community cohesion: A new framework for race and diversity*. Hampshire, UK: Palgrave Macmillan.

Champagne, E., 2009. Together on the journey of plurality. *International Journal of Children's Spirituality*, 14(1), pp. 1–3.

Davie, G., 2015. *Religion in Britain: A persistent paradox*. Oxford, UK: Wiley-Blackwell.

Davie, G., 2013. *The sociology of religion: A critical agenda*. London, UK: Sage.

Davie, G., 2007. Vicarious religion: A methodological challenge. In Ammerman, N.T. (ed.), *Everyday religion: Observing modern religious lives*. New York, NY: Oxford University Press, pp. 21–36.

Davie, G., 1994. *Religion in Britain since 1945: Believing without belonging (making contemporary Britain)*. Oxford, UK: Blackwell.

Day, A., 2010. Propositions and performativity: Relocating belief to the social. *Culture and Religion*, 11(1), pp. 9–30.

Dinham, A., 2015. Religious literacy and welfare. In Dinham, A. and Francis, M. (eds.), *Religious literacy in policy and practice*. Bristol, UK: Policy Press, pp. 101–112.

Dinham, A., 2012. *Faith and social capital after the debt crisis*. Hampshire, UK: Palgrave Macmillan.

Dinham, A., 2009. *Faiths, public policy and civil society: Problems, policies, controversies*. London, UK: Palgrave Macmillan.

Dinham, A. and Francis, M. (eds.), 2015. *Religious literacy in policy and practice*. Bristol, UK: Policy Press.

Erdozain, D., 2012. "Cause is not quite what it used to be": The return of secularization. *English Historical Review*, 127(525), pp. 377–400.

European Court of Human Rights, 2013. *New guidance for religion or belief*. Available at: https://www.echr.coe.int/Pages/home.aspx?p=home

Fallding, H., 1974. *The sociology of religion: An explanation of the unity and diversity in religion*. Ontario, Canada: McGraw-Hill Ryerson.

Fischoff, E., 1993. *The sociology of religion: Max Weber*. Boston, MA: Beacon Press.

Fonseca, L.M. and Testoni, I., 2011–2012. The emergence of thanatology and current practice in death education. *Omega: Journal of Death and Dying*, 64(2), pp. 157–169.

Ford, D. and Higton, M., 2015. Religious literacy in the context of theology and religious studies. In Dinham, A. and Francis, M. (eds.), *Religious literacy in policy and practice*. Bristol, UK: Policy Press, pp. 39–54.

Garces-Foley, K. (ed.), 2006. *Death and religion in a changing world*. New York, NY: M.E. Sharpe.

Gomes, B. and Higginson, I.J., 2008. Where people die (1974–2030): Past trends, future projections and implications for care. *Palliative Medicine*, 22(1), pp. 33–41.

Green, S.J.D., 2011. *The passing of Protestant England: Secularisation and social change, c.1920–1960*. Cambridge, UK: Cambridge University Press.

Guyau, J.M., 2015. *The nonreligion of the future: A sociological study*, vol. 39. New York, NY: Henry Holt.

Habermas, J., 2008. *Between naturalism and religion: Philosophical essays*. Malden, MA: Policy Press.

Habermas, J. and Seidman, S., 1989. *Jürgen Habermas on society and politics: A reader*. Boston, MA: Beacon.

Hansen, R., 2000. *Citizenship and immigration in postwar Britain*. Oxford, UK: Oxford University Press.

Hervieu-Léger, D., 2000. *Religion as a chain of memory*. New Brunswick, NJ: Rutgers University Press.

Jong, J., 2015. On (not) defining (non)religion. *Science, Religion and Culture*, 2(3), pp. 15–24.

Karpov, V., 2010. Desecularization: A conceptual framework. *Journal of Church and State*, 52(2), pp. 232–270.

Lee, L., 2012. Research note: Talking about a revolution: Terminology for the new field of nonreligion studies. *Journal of Contemporary Religion*, 27(1), pp. 129–139.

Luckmann, T., 1990. Shrinking transcendence, expanding religion? *Sociology of Religion: A Quarterly Review*, 51(2), pp. 127–138.

Martin, D., 2005. *On secularization: Toward a revised general theory*. London, UK: Ashgate.

Martin, D., 1978. *A general theory of secularization*. Oxford, UK: Basil Blackwell.

Mayo, M., 2005. *Global citizens: Social movements & the challenge of globalization*. London, UK: Zed Books.

Meister, C. (ed.), 2011. *The Oxford handbook of religious diversity*. New York, NY: Oxford University Press.

Moore, D.L., 2015. Diminishing religious literacy: Methodological assumptions and analytical frameworks for promoting the public understanding of religion. In Dinham, A. and Francis, M. (eds.). *Religious literacy in policy and practice*. Bristol, UK: Policy Press, pp. 27–38.

Moore, D.L., 2006. Overcoming religious illiteracy: A cultural studies approach. *World History Connected*, 4(1), p. 43.

NHS England, 2014. *NHS England's Actions for End of Life Care*. Available at: https://www.england.nhs.uk/wp-content/uploads/2014/11/actions-eolc.pdf

Norris, F.W., 2011. Religious demographics and the new diversity. In Meister, C. (ed.), *The Oxford handbook of religious diversity*. New York, NY: Oxford University Press, pp. 201–213.

Office for National Statistics, UK Census 2011, 2011. Available at: http://www.ons.gov.uk/ons/datasets-and-tables/index.html?pageSize=50&sortBy=none&sortDirection=none&newquery=religion&content-type=Reference+table&content-type=Dataset.

Office for National Statistics, 1977. *Guide to Census Reports*. Available at: http://www.visionofbritain.org.uk/census/Cen_Guide.

Pentaris, P., 2014. Religion, secularism, and professional practice. *Studia Sociologica*, 6(1), 99–109.

PEW Research, 2012. *The global religious landscape: A report on the size and distribution of the world's major religious groups as of 2010*. Washington, DC: Pew Research.

Portmann, A. and Plüss, D., 2011. Good religion or bad religion: Distanced church-members and their perception of religion and religious plurality. *Journal of Empirical Theology*, 24(2), pp. 180–196.

Prochaska, F., 2006. *Christianity and social service in modern Britain: The disinherited spirit*. Oxford, UK: Oxford University Press.

Prothero, S. and Kerby, L.R., 2015. The irony of religious illiteracy in the USA. In Dinham, A. and Francis, M. (eds.), *Religious literacy in policy and practice*. Bristol, UK: Policy Press, pp. 101–112.

Quack, J., 2014. Outline of a relational approach to 'nonreligion'. *Method & Theory in the Study of Religion*, 26(4–5), pp. 439–469.

Redington, F.M. and Clarke, R.D., 1951. The papers of the Royal Commission on Population. *Journal of the Institute of Actuaries*, 77(1), pp. 81–97.

Stackhouse, J.G.J., 2011. Religious diversity, secularization, and postmodernity. In Meister, C. (ed.), *The Oxford handbook of religious diversity*. New York, NY: Oxford University Press, pp. 239–249.

Taylor, C., 2007. *A secular age*. London, UK: The Belknap Press of Harvard University Press.

Timmins, N., 1995. *The five giants: A biography of the welfare state*. London, UK: Harper Collins.

Voas, D., 2009. The rise and fall of fuzzy fidelity in Europe. *European Sociological Review*, 25(2), pp. 155–168.

Voas, D. and Day, A., 2007. Secularity in Great Britain. In Kosmin, B.A. and Keysar, A. (eds.), *Secularism & secularity: Contemporary international perspectives*. Hartford, CT: ISSSC.

Warner, M., Van Antwerpen, J. and Calhoun, C. (eds.), 2010. *Varieties of secularism in a secular age*. Boston, MA: Harvard University Press.

Williams, R., 2006. Secularism, faith and freedom. *The Archbishop of Canterbury (23 November 2006)*. Available at: http://www.archbishopofcanterbury.org/654 and http://www.pass.va/content/dam/scienzesociali/pdf/acta13/acta13-williams.pdf.

Wilson, B., 1966. *Religion in secular society*. London, UK: C.A. Watts.

Weller, P. (ed.), 2007. *Religions in the UK: Directory 2007–2010*. Derby: University of Derby Press.

Wohlrab-Sahr, M., 2003. Politik und Religion: Diskretes Kulturchristentum als Fluchtpunkt europäischer Gegenbewegungen gegen einen ostentativen Islam [Politics and religion: A discrete cultural Christianity as the vanishing point of European counter-movements against an ostentatious Islam]. *Soziale Welt*, 14, pp. 357–381.

Woodhead, L. and Catto, R. (eds.), 2012. *Religion and change in modern Britain*. New York, NY: Routledge.

3 Tracing religion in health and death policy

Introduction

The task of observing, understanding and conceptualising the place of religion and belief in practise is not an easy one, however not impossible. To enable us to understand better the observations presented in the second part of the book, and which shed some light on this task, it is imperative also to look at the framework of social policy and appreciate how religion, belief and spirituality are embedded in it. This is where we now turn our attention.

The title of this chapter raises questions from the start. First and foremost, why health and death policies, and what are those policies? Next, what does the use of the term 'tracing' allude to? Last, what do we mean by social policy in general? This chapter discusses literature and policies which offer some answers to these questions, but neither widely nor exhaustively. Its main purpose is to provide enough information for readers to comprehend better the overall argument of this book.

Social policy is an integral part of social life – explaining the functional order of the latter. In general, social policy responds to concerns with principles about certain areas of social life, like religion and belief (Titmuss, 1974). Titmuss (1974, p. 138) suggests that policy refers to 'the principles that govern action directed towards given ends. The concept denotes action about means as well as ends and it, therefore, implies change: changing situations, systems, practices, behaviour'. In other words, policy has change in its core and aims at implementing change which will, in most cases (Alcock, 2014), constructively and positively enhance social life. Titmuss (1974), following on this suggestion, argues that social policy is only meaningful when society believes it can affect change. Alternatively, policy addresses areas over which people have power (e.g., professional practise), but not areas like natural disasters, as those are areas over which people have no control. This is a rather imperative conclusion as it identifies when policy is relevant, as well as that societies have either no power over social issues or phenomena which are not yet embedded in policy, or have not found a way in which to overpower them. This is relatively important to reminisce when examining the concept and traditions of religion in current policy; it leads to the question of whether religion is simply (even though not a simple question) overriding societies' ability to comprehend and control it, hence being unable to regulate it. As Titmuss (1974, p. 140) put it: 'social policy (or, to be more precise, a system of social welfare) is simply part of the self-regulatory mechanisms built into a "natural" social system'.

Conclusively, Titmuss (1974, p. 141) finds that 'social policy can be seen as a positive instrument of change; as an unpredictable, incalculable part of the whole political process'. Yet, despite its potential for positive outcomes, social policy is the tool by which change is implemented, and, therefore, it can be used in various ways and for various purposes. In particular, social policy does not always aim towards social welfare. There have been (and still are some) policies with purposes different from social welfare and the promotion of wellbeing. Titmuss offers a few examples, but the most evident is, perhaps, Hitler's social policies in Nazi Germany; those policies were not concerned with the welfare of people, for instance. Expressly, social policy does not always necessitate change towards equality nor is it concerned with altruism. Furthermore, Titmuss highlights that we should not think that current social policies in developed countries (e.g., Britain) always materialise in a way which ensures progression and equal opportunity for all. Titmuss (1974, p. 142) describes this well: 'What is "welfare" for some groups may be "illfare" for others'. Accepting the latter leads to the most important question: Whom is social policy for?

This discussion naturally leads us to think that social policy is not neutral of values; it often is a reflection of societal and individual principles and values; however, whose values are reflected in policy, and are any of them universal? Perhaps the answer to this question is conflicting or diffident. For example, Dombrowski (2001) quickly alluded to the conclusion that religion, among other personal characteristics, divides people, but social policy's aim is to offer more collective ways of bringing them together. This view is also influenced by Habermas' (2006) ideas about religion in the public sphere. Dombrowski (2001, p. 4) opines that 'pluralism has made religious liberty possible'; the greater the variety of religious traditions in societies, the more pressing the need to accommodate them. Equally, Habermas (2006) supports that policy became increasingly secular, especially in western societies, by means of neutral approaches to respond to religious plurality. To link these two positions to the question posed at the beginning of this paragraph: Does a neutral or secular or free-of-religious-conviction policy carry principles and values which are universal? According to Habermas (2006), the answer to this question is dubious.

The political philosopher John Rawls was influential to Habermas' arguments in various ways. Rawls' (1997) idea of public reason became fundamental in the exploration of the relationship between politics and religion. Since the 1990s, when issues of inequality became more important to social policy (Nesbitt, 2001), the latter's aim evolved into an all-inclusive way of responding to social issues informed by personal and collective identities.

Drawing on the idea of public reason, Habermas (2006) claimed that religion is embedded in religious people's political existence. Therefore, religious and political convictions intertwine, and a state of equilibrium between the two lies in the process of providing a logical and often traditional reasoning.

Complementary to this discussion is Weithman's (2002) argument that churches and religious organisations actively fulfil roles which promote and enhance the reproduction of democracy. Habermas (2006, p. 11) suggests that 'citizens of a democratic community owe one another good reasons for their political statements and attitudes'. Habermas (2006) focussed on the religious and nonreligious citizens' responsibility to sustain an open mind to the different views presented to them and identify truths in those presentations, which may enhance their political convictions.

In summary, social policy, among other purposes (also see Alcock, 2014), seeks to negotiate the multitude of attitudes, behaviours and characteristics in each society to promote its wellbeing and welfare, as well as its individual members. It is Habermas' (2006) view on mutual respect and Rawls' (1997; 1993) idea of public reason which inform the way in which this book incorporates social policy to its argument. The following sections look carefully at the way some key health and death policies (i.e., policies informing practise in end of life care) present religion, belief and spirituality. Such a process helps us 'trace' religion in this area and, therefore, appreciate when, how and under what circumstances identities related to faith are explored.

What policy says about religion and belief in dying

The tensions I have been exploring between religion and spirituality find expression in the policies which relate to the practise of care in death and dying settings. In this section, such policies are explored – primarily, the key legislation around EOL care in the UK.

Various disciplines are involved with EOL care delivery. EOL care is a wider field than just palliative care. Palliative care is an intervention that aims to eliminate pain and control symptoms (Saunders, 1992) and generally increase the presence of medicine and pathology in death, dying and bereavement (Walter, 1994). However, palliative care is one of the reasons why EOL care is embedded in social policy – moving forwards from an NHS that focusses on bio-medical approaches and enhances opportunities for the prolongation of life. The latter is also evident from the change of terms when discussing the care of the dying. The substitution of the term 'terminal care' with 'palliative care' in the 1980s was a milestone at a time when EOL care was leaning towards medicine and life-sustaining interventions (Walter, 1994). The NHS End of Life Care Programme 2004–2007, a programme launched in 2004, advances different than the bio-medical perspectives. The programme aimed to comprehend the need for future healthcare policies regarding EOL care and to set the boundaries between healthcare and palliative care. Predominantly, the objectives of the programme were to improve the quality of care at the end of people's lives and to enable more and more people to die at the place of their preference. Also, by the end of the programme, the intention was to develop services in end of life which would offer a much greater choice to people at the end of their lives. It would minimise the number of patient transfers from care homes to general hospitals during the last few days of their lives, and would enable generalist practitioners to familiarise themselves with EOL care models to improve the quality of care.

The programme materialised by means of three key practical solutions: the Gold Standards Framework (GSF), the Liverpool Care Pathway (LCP), and the Preferred Place of Care Plan (PPCP). The GSF is concerned with three main areas: identifying when people are near the end of their lives, assessing dying persons' needs, and recording persons' preferences. The LCP was developed from within hospice care, primarily for use in hospital settings where many people die, and is focussed on promoting good communication between families, patients and care staff. Last, the PPCP is a document that patients hold and which is used to record preferences, thoughts and desired place of death. These are a few key initiatives which indicate a shifting attitude in EOL care overall, and hospice care specifically, to record patient preferences and take them into account when planning care.

In 2008, 60 years after the establishment of the NHS, the first death policy was introduced, explicitly regarding EOL care: the End of Life Care Strategy 2008. Followed by a number of documents and complementary social policies and guidelines for EOL care (i.e., NHS Constitution in 2013, the LCP in 2009, End of Life Assessment annual documents, Better Care Better Lives 2008, to name a few), the emergence of the strategy acted as a milestone with regards to the care of dying adults. EOL care for children and young people is still a touchy subject and is less scrutinised in the UK. An important step towards the advancement of children's hospice care was offered by Children's Hospice UK and Together for Short Lives, in 2012.

The strategy is primarily led by the principles of the modern hospice movement; the document begins with a quote from Dame Cicely Saunders. This guidance goes beyond the care of symptoms and pain and intervenes towards the care of the psyche and psychosocial care. All patients, families and carers are involved in this strategy; however, it is focussed on the care of adults rather than children or minors. This is a death policy which was developed around the idea that people do not experience death or the dead body until at least midlife, and it reflects the fact that British society does not yet discuss death and dying openly and/or comfortably (Jupp and Howarth, 2016). It is specifically highlighted that health and social care staff fail to have discussions about the end of life (Department of Health, 2008, p. 23; Dillon, 2016), which makes social policy planning even more demanding.

End of Life Care Strategy 2008

The End of Life Care Strategy 2008 states that it is important to train healthcare professionals who practise in EOL care settings, like hospices, to identify dying people and initiate 'discussions about preferences for end of life care' (Department of Health, 2008, p. 11) – in other words, focus on *choice*. Borgstrom and Walter (2015) opine that since the strategy came into effect, two discourses have developed simultaneously: one about personal choice, which links with the conversations about advanced care planning, and the other about compassionate care. Both discourses are imperative in the renewed interest in spiritual care. The attention shifted in policy and care became more sensitive towards individual characteristics, like religion and belief.

Furthermore, there are two components of care in this report (Department of Health, 2008). First, professionals are expected to become more competent in their skills, abilities and values to accommodate better the imminent death of a person, and not push towards life-sustaining medication. The second part of the report encourages discussions about end of life and death, and appreciation and respect for dying people's preferences. This is challenging for workers simply due to the fear of one's own death, and will always be reminded of this by the death of the other (Kamath, 1993). Despite the challenge, the strategy suggests that patient preferences should be taken into consideration when planning and delivering care. Equally, professionals working in EOL care settings, according to the strategy, should further develop their skills and abilities to meet the needs of people when at the end of their lives, or near (also Department of Health, 2008, p. 17, §§1, 2, and 5). Healthcare professionals should have necessary skills and knowledge towards 'assessing needs' (Department of Health, 2008, p. 11), so that EOL care is addressed with inclusiveness and 'excellence' (also highlighted by the National Institute of Health and Care Excellence at http://www.nice.org.uk/).

Underlined in the End of Life Care Strategy 2008 is that healthcare professionals should have the 'right attitudes' and skills to develop practises appropriate and adequate to everyone who needs care (Department of Health, 2008, pp. 12–13). This is expected regardless of service users' personal characteristics such as culture, language, gender and religion, to name a few. The strategy refers to 'high quality services' (Department of Health, 2008, p. 13) in EOL care. Of great importance are the following: (1) in §19, the strategy suggests that a carer's care plan should always be in place as well, because 'carers might also have emotional needs'; (2) in §§20 and 21, considerations be given to what should be included in end of life care education; (3) provision of adequate training of staff and (4) provision of sufficient support for carers. It is on these four areas that social policy has largely focussed since, whereas practise has experienced some radical changes in the past decade – notably, excessive training of staff members – however filled with practical solutions, public awareness of hospice and palliative care and the more recent start of a dialogue about inequalities in EOL care. An example of a practical solution in practise is the way 'choice' has emerged in practise. Borgstrom and Walter (2015), among other scholars, identified this emergence as a tick-box exercise. Indeed, drawing on Pentaris (2016), choice is given to patients and their families, but only with the proviso that it is one of the options offered.

Noteworthy is that the UK strategy has adopted principles and priorities by EOL care strategies in Australia (2000), Canada (2000) and New Zealand (2001). All strategies had a special focus on identifying preferences towards the end of a patient's life, offering choice, as well as providing adequate resources to satisfy those preferences and promote quality services, as well as ensure a sense of equal opportunity in the services. Yet, what makes this remark important is the different contexts in which the principles apply. Drawing on Oliver's (1965) cultural flexibility – and the idea that principles and values are not universal, but specific to the environment in which they apply (or do not) – the UK strategy's challenge, among others, was to negotiate its aims, objectives and general intentions, as well as underpinning values, to fit the UK environment of EOL care.

Finally, and most importantly, the UK strategy in 2008, besides recognising patient preferences, encouraged the conversation about place of death. Both areas refer to the concept of *choice* and are linked directly with patients' cultural, religious and traditional backgrounds, which made the need to focus on religion and belief more pressing. However, given the changing place of religion and belief in society (see Chapter 2), spiritual care took hold in EOL care and acted as a proxy for religion and belief – a term (i.e., 'spiritual care') rather vague to represent a person's identity fully.

Spiritual care at the end of life

Chapter 1 discussed the place of spiritual care in hospice care extensively and offered information about the tensions between the vagueness of the term 'spiritual care' and its attempt to meet service user needs. This section focusses on a systematic review of the literature published by the Department of Health (Department of Health, 2009); it offers an in-depth account of how spiritual care should or is materialising in practise. With this account, this section identifies and offers a first degree of analysis regarding how 'religion', 'belief', 'spirituality' and/or other related terms appear in the review.

With abundant references to the hospice movement and Dame Cicely Saunders, the systematic review on spiritual care at the end of life (Department of Health, 2009) scrutinises hospice care and the responsibility for a holistic approach, including spiritual care for patients and carers. The authors of the report suggest that, due to deficiencies in service provision and professional practise, patients and/or carers may experience unnecessary spiritual suffering. The latter term, however, lacks description and definition, and thus is vague in interpretation. Despite the clear intentions of the meaning of spiritual suffering, the authors imply that emotions are included in spiritual care too, which might be; however, nowhere across the review is spiritual care explained or defined. On this note, and as spiritual care in EOL care appears to act as emotional and psychosocial care, this challenges the healthcare professionals' (inclusive of social care professionals in other than the UK context) roles and responsibilities (e.g., social work roles, psychology). Reminiscing Puchalski et al. (2009) and the report of the Consensus Conference about improving the quality of spiritual care in palliative care (discussed in Chapter 1), professional roles are blurred regarding who is responsible and for what, especially when discussing spirituality.

Attention is paid, in the review, to spiritual care for patients and their families, and there is a strong link between the care pathways – particularly the LCP. The sixth step in the LCP suggests that all staff be responsive to cultural, religious or spiritual needs. As with many other policy documents, these clustered needs are framed in an unruly and opaque way. It is advocated that people 'have spiritual, religious or emotional needs' (Department of Health, 2009, p. 75) – this being one of the only times the term 'religion' appears in the document. Before this section delves into examining the conceptual presence of religion-related terms in the document, it is important to remark that only the terms 'religion', 'spirituality' and 'faith' appear in the text.

Religion

Although both documents, *End of Life Care Strategy 2008* (Department of Health, 2008) and *Spiritual Care at the End of Life* (Department of Health, 2009), are circulating information with regards to respective attitudes towards diverse populations, high-quality hospice services and the need for spiritual care provision, the matter of religious beliefs is rarely introduced – or discussed. 'Spiritual/religious' needs are listed with the factors that influence needs and preferences of patients and family or friends (Department of Health, 2009, p. 45, §3.2). Table 3.1 notes the mentions of 'religion' and 'religious needs' in the document.

Table 3.1 offers an exhaustive list of the times when 'religion' is mentioned in the document (Department of Health, 2009). Expressly, 'religion' is mentioned 12 times and 'religion' is introduced in the following ways: in relation to organ donation, as an affiliation and with regards to demographics, and as an impacting factor on care, with limited expansion on the latter. Reference to religion in relation to organ donation, and perhaps handling of the body, is not surprising. Kellehear (2000) discussed a classification of spiritual needs in palliative and hospice care when he talked about the practical solutions offered. Pentaris (2016) also offers an exhaustive presentation of empirical knowledge verifying this in practise. Furthermore, showing interest to religion in terms of statistics and measurements may

Table 3.1 Systematic review: Mentions of 'religion' and 'religious needs'

'Religion'
• 'High quality care for all people approaching end of life should be irrespective of … religious belief and ethnicity' (p. 10, §7).
• 'high quality care for all people approaching end of life should be irrespective of … religious belief and ethnicity' (p. 33, §1.33).
• 'raising awareness of death and dying can also be taken forward by religious organisations. Those can promote understanding and information' (p. 39, §2.8).
• 'it is suggested that in the 6th step all staff should be responsive to cultural religious or spiritual needs' (p. 67).
• 'religious beliefs to be respected when it comes to organ donation' (p. 71, §3.83).
• 'body to be handled according to any religious beliefs' (p. 72, §3.84).
• 'disposal of the body: be aware of different religious perspectives' (p. 73, §3.85).
• 'Spiritual care services recognise that individuals may hold to a religious or non-religious belief system' (p. 75, §3.98).
• 'organization must obtain consent before sharing information on religious affiliation with chaplains' (p. 76, §3.102).
• 'Healthcare chaplains to have network of other religious ministers in the community' (p. 77, §3.105).
• 'religious competencies in all core training' (p. 77, §3.107).
• 'Religion and belief to be included in the demographics/stats collection' (p. 82, §4.11).

Source: Department of Health, 2009. *Spiritual care at the end of life: A systematic review of the literature.* London, UK: Department of Health.

also be expected, yet lacks in substance, with the intention being to improve quality of care, which requires excessive understanding of people's faith or lack of (Pentaris, 2012). Last, the review document (Department of Health, 2009) does not identify or explain what the impact on religion is on care, or how religion impacts on care. The document emphasises the importance of religion, but lacks depth in explanation and therefore leaves the text open to interpretation – vague and inaccessible.

Furthermore, the systematic review (Department of Health, 2009) refers to both spirituality and faith, often used interchangeably with the term 'religion'. This makes the process of identification and definition-giving a lot harder as it mixes meanings and concepts, that might as well be cultural-, religious- or person-specific. This indecisive attitude towards language, definition and concept is a struggle in itself. There are elements to it that go against the clarity of what religious creeds have historically offered: 'defence against death' (Walter, 1994, p. 14). Religious creeds have framed an afterlife in heaven and a well-developed exploration of the soul and eternity. References to spiritual care that includes religious needs, emotionality, psychosocial aspects of care and a general understanding of belief are merely not clear enough. Such a matrix offers countless contradictions and controversies, all of which are subject to further exploration.

Spirituality

Spiritual Care at the End of Life (Department of Health, 2009) is a 10-year literature review with the single aim to identify spiritual assessment tools, intervention models and general practises in EOL care settings. Therefore, the term 'spirituality' is used centrally in the document. Yet, the term is only mentioned a few times, in the proviso that the overall review is in the context of spiritual care.

Table 3.2 shows a few examples of when and how the term 'spirituality' is used in the systematic review. The report communicates, in all its length and broadly, that patients and family or carers have or may have spiritual needs. The reference to these needs, however, lacks definition or guidance for healthcare professionals to be well equipped to provide such services and meet those needs, but also be in the right place to measure the outcomes of service provision, towards the improvement and development of the services. This lack of definition was discussed in Chapter 1 and I return to it in Part II. Yet, it is important to mention, first, that the fuzziness of the term in policy and guidance documents is reflected in practise (see Chapters 5–7). Next, reminiscing Bregman's (2012) view that the term's obscurity may be purposeful, it may need to serve multiple purposes and this purpose may be disadvantaged if the term 'spirituality' is too specific.

Table 3.2 Systematic review: Mentions of 'spirituality'

'Spirituality'
• 'Over the past 40 years hospices … have demonstrated what can be done to provide physical, psychological, social and spiritual care for people and their families. Hospices are the good example of how to deliver qualitative spiritual care' (p. 7 forward).
• 'Due to deficiencies in service provision and professional practice, patients and/or carers may experience unnecessary spiritual suffering' (p. 24, §1.5).
• 'past work taught us that paying close attention to spiritual needs of patients and families, can improve end of life care' (Saunders' quote cited in source, p. 28, §1.16).
• 'Ensuring access to spiritual care' (p. 33, §1.34).
• 'Spiritual care is integral to the end of life care pathway' (p. 49, §3.13).
• 'spiritual dimension of each person' (p. 49, §3.99).
• 'Spiritual care is to allow the "person to express anger, guilt, sadness and reconciliation"' (p. 49, §3.100).
• 'Chaplains provide spiritual care to all staff as well' (p. 49, §3.101).
• 'spiritual competencies in core training' (p. 49, §3.107).
• 'Hospice care includes and always included spiritual care' (p. 95, §4.40).
• 'carers of the dying face spiritual consequences' (p. 107, §5.1).
• 'Staff providing bereavement services to family – after death – should have access to spiritual support' (p. 107, §5.18).

Source: Department of Health, 2009. *Spiritual care at the end of life: A systematic review of the literature.* London, UK: Department of Health.

Spiritual Care at the End of Life (Department of Health, 2009) also supports that hospices are the rightful institutions to be delivering spiritual care, and at the same time it is highlighted that each person has spiritual dimensions. Also, spiritual suffering is identified as the outcome of deficiencies in service provision or professional practise, whereas spiritual care is to offer to the individual the opportunity to express anger, sadness and guilt.

Interestingly, *Spiritual Care at the End of Life* (Department of Health, 2009) seems to emphasise the need to meet service user spiritual needs, and places the responsibility of either positive or negative outcomes of that on professionals in the field. However, when examining this on an organisational level, it is apparent that practise may be informed by policy, but is still driven by the specificities of an organisation or institution. In other words, the outcomes of spiritual care are not just dependent on individual professionals, but on a much more complicated relationship between organisational foundations, the organisation and professionals (we return to this point later in Part III).

This rather puzzling mixture of arguments raises numerous questions, as well as favours a challenging attitude towards policy planning around this area. If spiritual suffering is the result of poor service provision and professional practise in hospice care, is this why hospices are the right places to deliver spiritual care? Are hospices responsible for causing spiritual distress and then providing services to remedy the situation and comfort the patients? Is spiritual care simply an approach for the individuals to express their disappointment in the face of deficiencies of service provision and professional practise? All these questions and many more come to the surface considering the language used in *Spiritual Care at the End of Life* (Department of Health, 2009) and how it is used.

Equally important to note is policy's tendency to identify spirituality or a *spiritual self* in every person associated with hospice services and EOL care in general. This impulse seems controversial for the following reason. Attaching spiritual beliefs or needs to each service user, for example, suggests that regardless of their preferences, which may state no spirituality in this instance, they will still be treated in the proviso that they are spiritual. This is an awfully complicated concept to examine, but with the help of Dashtipour (2012) and the idea of the construction of social identity, it is easy to appreciate that people perceive themselves and whatever identity others attach to them in a way that shows their progression of becoming and not their state of being. In this sense, people who identify (or not) as spiritual recognise the process in which they are becoming spiritual. If their care plan is dependent on professionals' assumptions that each person is not only spiritual but also that spiritual needs can be operationalised and models of practise generalised, we run the risk of causing spiritual distress (as the systematic review of spiritual care suggests [Department of Health, 2009]) as opposed to offer comfort. This is but one of the challenges that the fuzziness of the term 'spirituality' may be causing.

Faith

Before we conclude with the *Spiritual Care at the End of Life* (Department of Health, 2009) document, it is worth looking at another term pertinent to our discussion about religion and belief. The term 'faith' is used in the document three times. Most importantly, what is mentioned in the review is that 'lenders of different faith groups were included in the consultation process' of the development of spiritual care in EOL care (p. 34, §1.36). The latter raises questions around the politics of planning a relevant policy. If the language used still seems Christian-centred or secular (also see Chapters 6 and 7 in this volume), how is the contribution of the different faith groups evident? What is meant by faith here? These are questions which we can only answer by assumption, but we can certainly claim that further research and examination are necessary.

This review (Department of Health, 2009) is of utmost importance to this book's argument as it depicts how religion and belief are reflected in practise. A year after the systematic review was completed, an action plan with equality objectives became effective. This plan is designed to influence front-line EOL care, nonetheless with no immediate effect.

Religion and belief in healthcare: A new design

In October 2012, the Department of Health published *Equality Objectives Action Plan* (EOAP; September 2012–December 2013). Only in recent decades have equality and diversity issues become major topics for social policy and politics. The EOAP's aim is to highlight the importance of deliberating the differences between majority and minority populations, however defined. An additional aim is to underline the recurrent limitations and strengths in current social policies across health and social care (Department of Health, 2012).

EOAP promotes three principles: better health, better care and better value for all (Department of Health, 2012). The Action Plan acccelerates a discussion and suggestions for fundamental changes within the health and social care system, with the latter being recognised for lacking in expertise on equity and equality issues. Derived from the EOAP, the Department of Health Business Plan 2012–13 (Department of Health, 2011) developed priority principles and strategies, all based on and in line with the NHS Equality Delivery System (EDS) goals: improved health outcomes, patient access and experience, inclusive leadership and empowered, engaged and included staff (Department of Health, 2012). Reminiscing the NHS End of Life Care Programme 2004–2007, the Business Plan is looking to develop further – or devise new, if necessary – strategies which promote the wellbeing of individuals and health equality.

For the business plan to be successful, NHS staff members from a variety of disciplines are required to participate fully in its recommendations (Department of Health, 2012). The Department of Health has since been working to 'ensure equitable policy-making and improved health outcomes' (Department of Health, 2012, p. 6). The new business plan also includes a supportive body: Public Health England (PHE). This body aims to collate all previous information and data from health and social care sectors to support equality in care and inclusive social policy-making. PHE assumed its responsibilities on 1 April 2013 and is working 'with stakeholders to promote good practise in dignity in care for all people' (Department of Health, 2012, p. 11). The importance behind this is the establishment of dignity as a key priority for the services in health and social care and the NHS in general (Department of Health, 2012). One of the latest documents of the PHE (2016), *Faith at the End of Life*, is a resource for professionals and commissioners in the community. The guide addresses faith in EOL care. This is the first time that social policy, and death policies, have addressed religion and belief by name, and not used the term 'spirituality' as a proxy to discuss it. Nevertheless, the main difference between this recent resource and previous policies and guidelines is that the former relates to work in the community whereas the latter address the issues within institutionalised care of the dying. Furthermore, embedded in the NHS Constitution 2013, the National End of Life Care Intelligence Network (NEoLCIN) promotes equality and equity in healthcare and end of life care for both dying and bereaved individuals.

Furthermore, one of the core principles of the EOAP is the better value of the services. The equality objective here is to 'ensure, as a system leader allocating and distributing funding, that the drive to increase value, efficiency and productivity across the health and care system considers the needs of all people with protected characteristics' (Department of Health, 2012, p. 13).

EOAP is not just an action plan, but a call for the reformation of the NHS. In the report (Department of Health, 2012), suggestions for new policies and a 'new system' are made; 'equality and diversity is prioritised in the design of the new system' (Department of Health, 2012, p. 15). Among others, with this report, the Department of Health recognises that inequalities within the NHS exist, and that a new design of the system is required – one which focusses on inclusive professional practise across health and social care – 'building and developing relationships with stakeholders including those that represent groups with protected characteristics as appropriate, in order to improve policy design and delivery' (Department of Health, 2012, p. 17). It is encouraging to witness an inclusive attitude by the Department of Health and the NHS, in the face of globalised communities, that offers opportunities for representatives from all subgroups of the community to have regular participation with the National Stakeholder Forum, which examines key issues in health and social care. This is known as the 'new policy partner system' and was put in place in March 2013.

Effective social policy remains a legislative idea based on past events and data until future events may prove it as such. The new design for the NHS, which celebrates minority groups in the community and adopts a further inclusive character to all in practise and service delivery, has yet to be fully assessed.

This information on equalities and diversity relates to this book in an indirect way, and nonetheless is necessary to mention. Equalities are part of the language in communicating religious plurality and the shifting needs associated with it. It is also the language used to interpret observations and explanations of secularity within a religiously plural environment, in social policy that can be well comprehended and established by healthcare.

A second key issue that is worth noting refers to the definition of 'personal characteristics'. Woodhead (2009), with her research report for the EHRC, identifies and prioritises issues associated with religious and secular matters in modern Britain. Religion has been included as an equality strand, and discrimination on the grounds of religion and belief has been denounced in recent years. The new design for health and social care services by the Department of Health refers to 'personal characteristics' but does not define or name any of them. It suggests including stakeholders from minority groups from within the community, but does not identify the minority groups. It refers to dignity for all people, regardless of background, but without clarification of what kind of 'backgrounds' were in mind when the report was generated. We can assume that 'personal characteristics', as framed within the new NHS design, refer to the equality strands recognised by the government, including religion and belief. I proceed based on this assumption.

This is a ground-breaking period for Britain – to start including religious matters in legislation and policy-making associated with healthcare and, consequentially, hospice and palliative care. However, belief is not a mere indication of religion or religious affiliation. Beliefs may also be nonreligious (see Chapter 2). The latter remains a matter of social policy and inclusion within health legislation.

Reference to the Action Plan (Department of Health, 2012) that affects healthcare provision overall was necessary to lay the foundations for a discussion of practises in hospice care and religious literacy. Kübler-Ross (1972), in her discourse on a death-denying society, repeats the question: 'Why is dying different now?' (p. 174). People still hold the same subconscious thoughts on death and dying experiences. However, society is ever changing, alongside the settings that develop and deliver services to dying and/or bereaved systems. It is important, in consideration of providing quality services within the NHS, to have ensured first that the delivery system follows on successfully in light of the changes that globalisation, modernisation and secularisation bring to communities and larger societies (Meister, 2011). Shifting demographics signal the need for policy planning and organising according to shifting needs in the community. This book does not directly deal with changes in the composition of society. However, given these changes, and in particular the diversity observed in terms of religion and belief (Weller, 2007), we may ask whether we still possess the right language for the purposes of having this discussion in policy and practise.

Concluding thoughts

The ambiguity of the presentation of religion in social policy reminisces Audi's (2005) concept of a theo-ethical equilibrium. Audi explored how religious reasons may find place in a liberal state where secular ideas predominate. In his exploration, he argued that people of faith need to find a balance between both their religious and secular convictions. Along the same lines, the language used in social policy to discuss religion and belief remains vague, but perhaps with purpose. The 'open to interpretation' use of the term 'spirituality' is claimed to allow a wider set of identities to be discussed under its umbrella, which projects some of Audi's secular convictions. Simultaneously, policy, very recently (specifically, PHE, 2016), attempted to discuss religion explicitly and draw on identified religious traditions when setting guidelines towards improving the quality of services in EOL care in the community. It is the balance between the two which is most important and which remains a mystery to be solved. Currently, especially with recent government documents like *One Chance to Get It Right* (Department of Health and Social Care, 2014), *Our Commitment to You for End of Life Care* (Department of Health, 2016) and *One Year On: The Government Response to the Review of Choice in End of Life Care* (Department of Health, 2017), the intention remains to eradicate inequalities in EOL care while emphasising *compassionate care*.

In conclusion, the discussion returns to Titmuss (1974) and the question: *Whose social policy?* Policy is underpinned with principles and values, has specific intentions and leads to explicit outcomes. The latter is impacted by the two former, as well as the way it is interpreted and applied in practise. However, whose principles and values inform policy planning? Under what circumstances? And, for whom is policy implemented? Expressly, whose benefits does it promote? This chapter may not offer an answer to these questions, but it draws attention to the ambiguity of policies in EOL care, healthcare, and hospice care specifically, while it identifies gaps in this area.

References

Alcock, P., 2014. *Social policy in Britain*. London, UK: Palgrave Macmillan.

Audi, R., 2005. Moral foundations of liberal democracy, secular reasons, and liberal neutrality toward the good. *Notre Dame Journal of Law, Ethics, & Public Policy*, 19, pp. 197–218.

Borgstrom, E. and Walter, T., 2015. Choice and compassion at the end of life: A critical analysis of recent English policy discourse. *Social Science & Medicine*, 136, pp. 99–105.

Bregman, L., 2012. Spirituality definitions: A moving target. In Fowler, M., Martin III, J.D. and Hochheimer, J.L. (eds.), *Spirituality: Theory, praxis, and pedagogy*. Oxford, UK: Inter-Disciplinary Press, pp. 3–10.

Dashtipour, P., 2012. *Social identity in question: Construction, subjectivity, and critique*. London, UK: Routledge.

Department of Health, 2017. *One year on: The government response to the review of choice in end of life care.* Available at: https://www.gov.uk/government/uploads/system/uploads/attachment_data/file/645631/Government_response_choice_in_end_of_life_care.pdf.

Department of Health, 2016. *Our commitment to you for end of life care: The government response to the review of choice in end of life care.* Available at: https://www.gov.uk/government/publications/choice-in-end-of-life-care-government-response.

Department of Health, 2012. *Equality objectives action plan.* London, UK: Department of Health.

Department of Health, 2011. *Department of Health Corporate Plan 2012-2013.* London, UK: Department of Health.

Department of Health, 2009. *Spiritual care at the end of life: A systematic review of the literature.* London, UK: Department of Health.

Department of Health, 2008. *End of life care strategy: Promoting high quality care for all adults at the end of life.* London, UK: Department of Health.

Department of Health and Social Care, 2014. *One chance to get it right: Improving people's experience of care in the last few days and hours of life.* Available at: https://www.gov.uk/government/publications/liverpool-care-pathway-review-response-to-recommendations.

Dillon, E.C., 2016. How home hospice care facilitates patient and family engagement. *Death Studies*, 40(10), pp. 591–600.

Dombrowski, D.A., 2001. *Rawls and religion: The case for political liberalism.* Albany, NY: State University of New York Press.

Habermas, J., 2006. Religion in the public sphere. *European Journal of Philosophy*, 14(1), pp. 1–25.

Jupp, P.C. and Howarth, G. (eds.), 2016. *The changing face of death: Historical accounts of death and disposal.* London, UK: Springer.

Kamath, M.V., 1993. *Philosophy of life and death.* Mumbai, India: Jaico Publishing.

Kellehear, A., 2000. *Experiences near death: Beyond medicine and religion.* Brisbane, Australia: Replica Books.

Kübler-Ross, E., 1972. On death and dying. *Journal of the American Medical Association*, 221(2), pp. 174–179.

Meister, C. (ed.), 2011. *The Oxford handbook of religious diversity.* New York, NY: Oxford University Press.

Nesbitt, P.D. (ed.), 2001. *Religion and social policy.* Oxford: AltaMira Press.

Oliver, S.C., 1965. Individuality, freedom of choice, and cultural flexibility of the Kamba. *American Anthropologist*, 67(2), pp. 421–428.

Pentaris, P., 2016. *Religious literacy in end of life care: Challenges and controversies.* Unpublished Doctoral Thesis (Goldsmiths, University of London).

Pentaris, P., 2012. Religious competence in social work practice: The UK picture. *Social Work & Society*, 10(2), pp. 1–4.

Public Health England, 2016. *Faith at the end of life: A resource for professionals, providers and commissioners working in communities.* London, UK: Department of Health.

Puchalski, C., Ferrell, B., Virani, R., Otis-Green, S., Baird, P., Bull, J., Chochinov, H., Handzo, G., Nelson-Becker, H., Prince-Paul, M. and Pugliese, K., 2009. Improving the quality of spiritual care as a dimension of palliative care: The report of the Consensus Conference. *Journal of Palliative Medicine*, 12(10), pp. 885–904.

Rawls, J., 1997. The idea of public reason revisited. *The University of Chicago Law Review*, 64, pp. 765–807.

Rawls, J., 1993. *Political liberalism*. New York, NY: Columbia University Press.

Saunders, C., 1992. Voluntary euthanasia. *Palliative Medicine*, 6(1), pp. 1–5.

Titmuss, R.M., 1974. *Social policy*. London, UK: Allen & Unwin.

Walter, T., 1994. *The revival of death*. New York, NY: Routledge.

Weithman, P.J., 2002. *Religion and the obligations of citizenship*. Cambridge: Cambridge University Press.

Weller, P. (ed.), 2007. *Religions in the UK: Directory 2007–2010*. Derby: University of Derby Press.

Woodhead, L., 2009. *"Religion or belief": Identifying issues and priorities*. London, UK: AHRC/ESRC Religion and Society Programme, Lancaster University.

Part II

Negotiating belief in hospice care

.

4 Belief in the space

Introduction

The exploration of belief – how it manifests itself in a single institution and how this manifestation is facilitated by policy and the organisational culture of the institution – is a multifaceted task that requires attention from various angles. When examining how religion, belief and spirituality are integrated aspects of professional practise and hospice care, it is imperative to consider how belief generally is represented in the space. Drawing on McGuire's (2008) work, this chapter is concerned with the lived religion of the hospice; it explores how belief is manifested and lived in hospices. McGuire (2008) was indeed more interested in the embodiment of spirituality and provides a sociological exploration of that; yet, he invoked further the issue of materiality and religion in everyday life (Keane, 2008), which directly influenced the dialogue in the sociology of religion about how and when religious or nonreligious beliefs become visible (Ammerman, 2016).

There have been but few studies exploring the material presence or absence in the space, unless in the arts and humanities (e.g., Horovitz, 2017). One example is that of Cadge and Konieczny (2014). These two scholars of palliative care explored the presence of religion in secular organisations. They used the term 'secular' more loosely to include nonreligious organisations as well. Their study aimed at examining how religion is lived out in such organisations and they concluded that this area remains grey, as the secular character of organisations is not always compatible with the beliefs of the people in the organisation. Another example is that of Kellehear, Pugh and Atter (2009), who carried out a photoethnography to examine bedside objects in a hospice, inclusive of religious objects, as discussed in the next section.

With this in mind, to comprehend better the complexity of how professionals respond to needs related to religion, belief and spirituality, it is necessary to look at how such topics are addressed in the space, which then helps with the progression of an understanding of the former. Of course, this task does not come without challenges. The main challenge considered in this chapter is also one of the main reasons that makes this chapter so important. There is a contextual challenge: When exploring a hospice in a single religious context, it is easy to address the question of the presence of that religion in the space. However, *what does the presence or obsolescence of one religion or another tell us when the hospice runs within a multi-faith environment?* We return to this question at the end of this chapter and the end of this book, as it brings rise to a key challenge that hospice care is facing nowadays. In the meantime, it is worth noting that I approach this question, throughout this chapter, from an anthropological viewpoint; the chapter grasps 'local knowledge' as explained by Clifford Geertz (1983).

Religion and materiality

The relationship between religion and materiality is a contested subject (Insoll, 2009). The essence of this discussion is about how religion and belief speak through practises, images and other material objects. However, such a notion contests what constitutes a material object, as well as what objects are of religious or nonreligious character. Furthermore, the use of religious icons, for example, helps make sense of belief but also evidences the culture which sustains such belief. Material religion, in other words, can be examined as to how it represents and expresses hospice and professional attitudes towards belief (Insoll, 2009). Similarly, Miller (2005, p. 2) suggests that 'humans are defined by their expressions of immaterial ideals through material forms'. Equally, material forms in the hospice or used by professionals are such expressions.

Morgan (1999, p. xi) explicitly argued that taking this into consideration when researching religion and belief is important 'because there is something irresistible about the fact that human consciousness owes so much to cardboard icons and plastic buttons'. Icons or crosses that mark the halls and rooms of a hospice, or are worn by hospice professionals, add to our understanding of the everyday life of the organisation. Both the presence and absence of religious objects and religious representations in the hospice in general add to the construction of social reality. How do professionals, patients, family members and friends, or visitors experience the hospice and the latter's relationship with faith? In other words, how does the hospice respond to faith?

In addition, the presence or absence of such objects demonstrates how a hospice accommodates needs related to religion, belief and spirituality. Such an example is shown by Kellehear, Pugh and Atter (2009). These scholars made connections between the objects that hospice patients kept at their bedside and what they meant to them. Despite the very few objects of religious significance that the authors observed, they enhanced the patient's sense of belonging and, both mentally and physically, reshaped the environment to accommodate better their psychoemotional and spiritual needs.

In the following two sections, I address two main themes: images and dress – in other words, the presence and absence of religious icons and other images of religious significance in a hospice. Second, I examine how professionals wear religious symbols whilst in practise. Both sections are informed by my fieldwork in hospice care. Last, the discussion in these sections materialises in the understanding that social policy governs professional practise (also see Chapter 3).

Images

There is scarce information available about the representation of faith in hospices via images. Research has long overseen the presence or absence of images in hospices, but targeted the meaning personal objects have for patients and their families and friends (Kellehear, Pugh and Atter, 2009). The latter is an exploration of religious materiality on the micro level – otherwise, individual. What about the macro level, though – the organisational?

From October 2013 to April 2015, I spent a significant number of hours per week making observations of whether, when and how religion, belief and spirituality are expressed via religious images in two very large hospices in the Greater London area. This period allowed me the opportunity to experience first-hand the changes that the hospices faced and how that led to a more neutral and free-from-religious-representations environment. This knowledge was later presented to hospice professionals across the Greater London Area in the UK, who provided feedback and consultation.

Until recently, in 2013, hospices still projected much of their religious history, and many religious icons adorned various parts of the hospices; crucifixes, crosses and framed religious texts decorated the walls of the corridors, offices, patient rooms, prayer and quiet rooms, the garden and the entrances. To exemplify the frequency with which one would come across a religious icon, more than 20 icons of Jesus Christ or Virgin Mary and baby Jesus adorned the corridors of each hospice. Large crucifixes were set in the lobby areas of the hospices and various small crosses were carefully placed in small dents in the wall when walking up and down the stairs. Furthermore, every prayer/quiet room was equipped with at least one crucifix and two icons with either Jesus Christ or the Virgin Mary and baby Jesus on them.

The use of images, crosses and crucifixes in the various spaces of a hospice can tell us a lot about its history, development and current character. Morgan (1999) has best argued this through the lens of history and culture; he maintains that to understand better the meaning and use of popular religious images, we first ought to understand what historians do. In other words, a better understanding of the history of religious images would enhance our appreciation of their contemporary presence. It is religious images that contribute to the construction of reality of the person, group or institution. Equally, the use, as well as how they are used, of religious images in a hospice show how the institution makes and sustains its reality, which then is projected or influences professionals and service users alike.

With this in mind, at the start of my exploration of how religion, belief and spirituality are expressed in hospices, on an organisational level, various religious objects adorned the various spaces. This made, however, an impression which was soon to change. Throughout my study (Pentaris, 2016), hospices saw a series of changes, whereas others impacted on single hospices. Regardless, such changes are reflected in a recent report by Hospice UK (2016) and often projected the intention of hospices to become more inclusive and expand the delivery of their services across the palette of ethnicities and religious (and nonreligious) beliefs in their communities. The most appropriate example is the April 2013 NHS Mandate, as well as the following document December 2014 NHS Mandate, which recognises the importance of EOL care (inclusive of hospice care) and suggests that inviting spaces, neutral of personal characteristics and preferences, should be a priority (Department of Health, 2014). The Enhancing the Healing Environment project is another reflection of this: a programme commissioned by the Department of Health and carried out by The King's Fund. The project's aim was to have professionals and service users work in partnership to develop the environment in which patients receive care (more information at https://www.kingsfund.org.uk/projects/enhancing-healing-environment).

Suggestions include the need to develop a physical environment in hospice care which is inviting to all cultures and religions. Therefore, the intent of the Mandate is that the internal and external of the hospices should remain neutral in terms of decorations and representations of particular cultures and/or religions. The opposite is considered to work towards excluding people from other religious groups or denominations, whereas the hope is to be inclusive. During my study, I spoke with various professionals in the hospices I observed and I collected stories which often highlight the necessity for this measure. An example is Camila, a 52-year-old nurse who said, 'We had a lady who [was] very reluctant to come here because there are nuns and, you know, crucifixes and rosaries and other stuff about Christianity'. This quote may indeed justify the measurements put in place with the Mandate, but it questions the liability and truthfulness of the measures. Are people reluctant due to an obviously open environment on religion and belief, or might it be due to a Christian-centred presentation of the institution? Are people of other than Christian faiths reluctant or everyone? What are people reluctant of? Dearth of data does not allow us to answer these questions yet, which raises another issue: How is the decision for neutral spaces made when there is no evidence to support that the opposite is what promotes ambivalence and inequality?

Moreover, recent research in children's hospice care has shown that a hospice religious character is not necessarily a barrier for preventing people from using the services (Pentaris et al., 2018). One of the most prominent reasons (but not a barrier) that stops people from making use of hospice care is their religious and cultural background (Yancu, Farmer and Leahman, 2010). Some cultures or religious traditions promote a very close-knit family system which then takes responsibility for the care of another family member towards the end of their life.

In the project by Pentaris (2016), by December 2014, in the attempt to neutralise the institution's character, a significant number of religious icons, crosses and crucifixes had been removed from hospice spaces (wards, halls, patient rooms, entrance of the hospice). This evidence is projected in more recent research by Walker and Breitsameter (2017). These two scholars explored the provision of spiritual care in four hospices in the most popular state of Germany: North Rhine-Westphalia. Their work partially looked at what religious items are used to decorate patient rooms, the entrance of hospices or the halls. Their research reported that the hospices were intentionally trying to avoid adorning the walls of the hospice with religious images or crosses, but if an image was used it would be one reflecting a *spiritual aspect of humanity* which could apply to all and not just one religious denomination.

The intentional absence of religious images, crosses, crucifixes or other items is impactful on various levels, which are explored in this book. Most relevant to this volume's argument is that spatial changes of this kind impact on professionals as well as the organisation (Bissell, 2012). Professionals, specifically, have started adjusting to the reason behind the obsolescence of religious items generally in hospices – in other words, developing ambivalence towards religion and belief, as we see later in this book, and suppressing the expression of their own faith to project professionalism.

Case study

Alex is a 55-year-old nurse who started working at the hospice 11 years ago. He accepted this job as his personal and religious values matched those of the hospice. For the first nine years, Alex was comfortable with the presence of the nuns in the hospice and the afternoon prayers on the wards. Alex joined the nuns to pray for patients' wellbeing; they would visit the different rooms and would either overtly or covertly pray for the patient's wellbeing. Only recently, have the nuns stopped visiting patients in their rooms, and afternoon prayers are not acceptable, as is not praying for the patients in their rooms. This change coincided with all religious images in the hallway being removed and the prayer room being designated a quiet room.

- *How could these changes affect Alex's practise, if at all? On what level?*
- *How could these changes impact public perceptions about how hospice care responds to religion, belief and spirituality?*

Dress

One way of exploring how religion, belief and spirituality are projected in hospices and on an organisational level is by looking at how professionals wear religious symbols. Hospice and palliative professionals represent the organisation's character, appearance and attitude. Patients, family members, friends or the general public often appreciate hospices and hospice care through the actions or inactions of professionals (Csikai, 2006). To a certain extent, professionals are a living and moving canvas of the hospice. Professional attitudes and integrity are influenced by the organisational culture in which practise happens. Therefore, examining how professionals in hospices wear or do not wear religious symbols is a natural progression from our previous section on images in the space.

The difficulty in determining what constitutes a religious symbol (Evans, 2008) is the main challenge in the task at hand. The exploration of how professionals wear religious symbols is unrealistic if we do not agree on what those symbols look like and what they are. In the *Manual on the Wearing of Religious Symbols in Public Areas*, Evans (2008) examines this challenge very carefully. Drawing on case laws and various conflicts involving religion and belief and human rights, Evans questions to whom is a religious symbol of religious significance, and how do we know whether it is for the state or the individual to determine the former. There is immense value in this, especially when using ethnographic research methods. The dichotomy of objectivity and subjectivity becomes highly relevant. Are there measurements to determine religious symbols or is it the person's responsibility to identify a symbol as religious to them? Wearing an item traditionally known as a religious symbol (e.g., headscarf) does not necessarily make the symbol religious, according to Evans (2008). Whether the person wearing the headscarf manifests their religion and belief through the headscarf is of importance (also see Mazzas, 2009).

> Perhaps surprisingly, the real significance of something being a religious symbol lies in the response of others to that symbol.... For example, not every turban or headscarf, cross, knife or bracelet has a religious significance for the wearer. Such objects might, however, have a religious significance for someone else who might consider their use or display by non-believers to be offensive. (Evans, 2008, p. 66)

This quote further highlights the two dimensions of the aforementioned challenge: the wearer's interpretation of what is religious and what is not, and a third party's perception about whether a symbol worn by someone is religious. This section takes these points very seriously and only discusses worn religious objects: Those which were identified and defined by those wearing them. The section also reflects on what reactions the wearers of religious symbols have gathered from patients and their families and friends.

An additional point made by Evans (2008) is that not all religious objects or symbols can be worn; some may be simply objects of religious significance to professionals which adorn the space and are not part of their attire. In other words, professionals also act as mediators of religious symbolism in hospices, between themselves and the hospice space.

Very often, religious symbols that are worn in public, aside from a head-scarf (Howard, 2013), are religious jewellery, like a cross around one's neck or on a bracelet. Research on religion and workplace has explored this widely, especially in light of the recent case of *Eweida and Others vs the United Kingdom* (Vickers, 2016), among others. Ms Eweida, a British Airways employee, was at the end denied permission to wear a cross around her neck at work. This example, aside from other things, shows us the public and legal intention to emphasise matters related to the wearing of religious symbols. The outcomes of such cases may also indicate general rules about how employees are expected to manifest their faith and whether health and safety issues arise from that. Otherwise, religious jewellery and how, when and why they are worn and shown or hidden in the workplace is also a subject impacted by European court cases on the grounds of religion and belief. Some lessons from how such cases influence professional behaviour may be transferable to hospice and end of life care, more generally (Treviño, Butterfield and McCabe, 1998). However, we have very little to no knowledge about how hospice professionals wear religious jewellery and the impact such representations have in practise. Pentaris (2016) focused on this and noted the shifting attitudes of professionals.

During the course of 18 months, and in the space of two large, urban hospices, only nine people were observed to wear one or more religious symbols. Specifically, professionals only wore religious jewellery, but adorned their workstations/desks with other items, such as small religious icons. Religious jewellery was discreetly worn by the staff and was gently covered with a part of their clothing – such as a sleeve – when entering a patient's room, especially if the patient was known to be of different faith than the professional's. Hospice professionals from various disciplinary backgrounds, including nursing, medicine and occupational therapy, are indeed challenged to find the proper balance between three aspects influencing their practise: professionals' personal faith and how they wish to express it, the organisational culture and how faith is projected or expected or not to be projected on that level, and how either of these two aspects, or their interaction, impact the service user experience.

Some scholars have considered, especially in nursing (Stephenson, Draucker and Martsolf, 2003), that spiritual care has been largely neglected in hospice care. The fine line, though, between neglect and illiteracy is gaunt and easily crossed. The hiding of religious jewellery before entering a patient's room can be interpreted in various ways. Drawing on Pentaris (2016), professionals stated at large that they find it the least challenging to provide services to individuals with different faiths from theirs, given that their faith is important to them. The general practise observed was that professionals would reveal their religious jewellery once they had left the patient's room. In further discussions, it became evident that aside from the feelings of unease when working with individuals with a faith different from their own, hospice professionals are constantly trying to find a balance between their practise and either legislation or organisational policies. I do argue in this book that spiritual care has never been neglected. On the contrary, social policies, education and organisational contexts may have neglected to equip professionals fully to be able to deliver it. This is where the concept of religious literacy, despite its unsteady definition (also see Chapter 2), as we see in Conclusions at the end of this book, becomes relevant; lack of religious literacy results in professionals being unable to address religion, belief and spiritual identities of their patients and thus come across as neglectful. A perfect reflection of this is seen in Sue and Sue (2012). They stated that cultural competence has become paramount in professional practise since the beginning of the new millennium. Since, literature argues that lack of cultural competence may present itself as neglect in professional practise (Johnson et al., 2004). Nonetheless, it is still unclear whether professionals are projected as neglectful or whether policy and organisational culture transform practise as mediated through professionals into neglectful.

By and large, hospice professionals have received training and guidance by hospice organisations in the UK to best avoid engaging with religion-, belief- and spirituality-related matters. The general advice is to employ a most neutral attitude towards these matters – advice that is naturally expected when revisiting NHS Mandate 2014, discussed earlier in this chapter. Professionals involved in my project (Pentaris, 2016) stated that their respective hospice organisations have directly been instructed to promote an open and inclusive environment, which can only be achieved by avoiding reference to specific religions.

This discussion triggers numerous questions. Some very important ones are the following: Are current trends in practise at the expense of the professionals and service users? How far do neutrality and impartiality promote and enhance the wellbeing of service users or accommodate needs as they emerge from the rapidly changing demographics of the population? Debates about ideas of the secular are directly linked with the neutral stance that professional practise is promoting. Sue and Sue (2012) explored the oppressive feelings of people with different characteristics to highlight, on the one hand, the importance of cultural competence (including religion), but on the other, that cultural competence involves self-understanding and self-awareness of the professional. Cultural competence is embraced not by hiding one's true characteristics but by remaining true to the service user and, therefore, having rapport and an honest and open communication.

When looking at both the general space (e.g., wards, corridors, entrance of a hospice) and how professionals in that space wear or do not wear religious symbols, we can reach the unmistakable conclusion that one is the extension of the other. In other words, when professionals attempt to hold on to their wearing of a bracelet, it almost feels like a rebellious act. It is an action that causes distress to the professional and that later is projected on their practise. Unfortunately, this is as far as this argument can go, due to lack of further evidence, yet I argue that there is reason to explore further the counter-impact of not wearing religious symbols, when wanting to, on service users; and eventually on their wellbeing.

Case study

Sometime around midnight, a patient pulled the emergency cord in his room. I got up and made my way to the room as quickly as possible. In the meantime, I thought about who that patient was – a 76-year-old man without many family members, who specified when he arrived that he is Muslim. We offered him all the options available for Muslims, but he did not always accept them. As I got closer to the room, I thought that I did not want to upset him because of the cross I wear around my neck. I quickly tucked that inside my blouse and entered the room. I untucked it when I went out.

- *How does the professional feel about having to tuck in her cross before entering the patient's room?*
- *Did she need to tuck the cross inside her blouse? Why? Why not?*
- *Are there any underpinning assumptions in the professional's behaviour?*

Religion and belief in the space

Religion and belief are either present or absent in various ways in hospices. In the following sub-sections, I tell a story about how religion, belief and spirituality have been accommodated in the hospice on an organisational level. This story begins with chapels and progresses towards how service users make use of the outdoor space of a hospice – in this case, a garden. This narrative also presents the transformation of prayer rooms into something different and with a different purpose.

Chapel

Chapels have been an integral part of hospices since the 19th century (Winslow and Clark, 2005). The functions of a chapel have, for a long period, been compatible both with the way hospice care was conceptualised in the mid-20th century by Cicely Saunders (also see Chapter 1), but also with the hospice philosophy in the 20th century. Parkes' (1979) work, among others', illustrates this. In an exploration of how bereaved individuals appreciated in-patient services at St Christopher's Hospice, Parkes (1979) found that patients were aware of chapel services and the majority were glad of them.

Following the developments of care in the 1990s, the role of chapels was revisited (VandeCreek and Burton, 2001). The debates about spiritual care and how to locate religion in it was of great significance, and still is. It became imperative, given the increasing religious diversity of the population (see Chapter 2), that professional chaplains engage in activities beyond the space of a chapel (VandeCreek and Burton, 2001). Hence, even though chapels continued to open during the 1990s (29% of all chapels), in both hospitals and hospices, multi-faith rooms were popularised (91% of all multi-faith rooms) (Wright, 2001). The intention to widen the scope of the services and promote impartiality led to a less chapel-orientated approach. Nevertheless, chapels remain open in hospices (children's or not). If spiritual care is relocated to multi-faith rooms, or quiet rooms as we see later, what are chapels used for, apart from the Mass?

During my study (Pentaris, 2016), only one (out of two) of the chapels was open, yet not throughout the whole period. The first nine months during which participant observation was taking place, the chapel of the hospice had been closed due to renovations. For nine months, people would follow the signs to the chapel and then encounter a large sign which read that renovations were taking place. People were informed they could start visiting the chapel after June 2014; I did. I first describe my experience and then discuss it more extensively.

The chapel is located in the building where all the business components of the hospice are and it took good physical health to get there; as there is, for example, no lift, but only stairs. The interior of the chapel is not dissimilar than elsewhere; there are religious wall murals and a large crucifix in the centre and numerous prayer benches around the room. When one enters on the right-hand side, there is a bench with bibles for public use while at Mass. All this is as expected and indicates the chapel is still in use, accommodating people's Christian needs. Of course, in this case, only people with the physical ability to reach the chapel can benefit from the services.

Moreover, the services in the chapel are hour-specific. Chapels in hospices have opening hours. Reminiscing Cadge's (2013) argument for on-call spiritual carers, the chapel here is not an on-call service (even though chaplains often carry beepers to come in and provide spiritual care when and where necessary [Wright, 2001]). People who wish to make use of space in the chapel, though, need be aware of the opening hours and schedule their visit accordingly. This depicts a comforting situation when one has no urgency to pray or seek any other form of spiritual support (Cadge, 2013) and, therefore, can schedule their visit.

Another important finding is the following. When entering the chapel, on the left-hand side, there is space for artists with an interest in Christianity. In this space, artists can exhibit and sell their work. The usage of the chapel diversified and it became more than a space for worship, prayers and religious practise. It reopened and offered an additional opportunity for merchandise and product exchange, as well as fundraising opportunities. This is somewhat oppositional to the architectural principles of a hospice building (McGann, 2013). McGann (2013) recommends that the building of the hospice needs to match hospice ideology; hence, to reflect an anti-institutional and anti-business character. However, it is apparent that even if the architecture of the building suggests differently, the way space is used indicates its purpose – in this case, a chapel is used both for worship and sales.

The 'showing' and 'selling' of art projects in the chapel also leads to the following conceptions. First, a chapel is presented as a touristic attraction, one that people would visit and buy a souvenir on their way out. Next, hospices are institutions that promote wellbeing and provide EOL care and, therefore, offer the opportunity for people to express their beliefs, fears and hopes in the chapel. Nonetheless, the exchange of products defeats the purpose as it contradicts the practise of neutral spaces. If people buy a religious icon, they are likely to display that in their room or relative's room. However, they are not encouraged to do so as the space, as discussed earlier, should be neutral and welcoming to all. The following case study represents this endless loop and invites readers to reflect on its various dimensions.

Case study

While feeling overwhelmed with the recent news about my husband – his condition got worse; the doctor cannot do anything but try and keep him comfortable – I decided to take some time off and sit quietly with my thoughts. I needed this to carefully think what his imminent death might mean. I decided to walk to the chapel. It should be quiet there and I can take as much time as I wish. When I walked in, a gentleman was speaking to a staff member from the cleaning services, a middle-aged lady was sitting on a bench quietly staring at the crucifix in front of her, lost in her thoughts, and another gentleman by the entrance was setting up a booth with rosaries with a tiny price sign next to them reading '£7 each, two for £10'.

- *What are your first impressions from this scenario?*
- *How many functions of the chapel can you identify in this scenario?*
- *Who may be disadvantaged in this scenario and why?*

Returning to Wright's (2001) work, chapels became of less interest in the everyday life of a hospice. As more modern ideas emerged and the diverse religious identities of patients raised the demands for appropriate care and response, multi-faith rooms seemed far more suitable for this purpose. This tension, the distancing of Christian spaces from the concept of spiritual care, is the aftermath of the separation of religion from spirituality. Bradshaw best describes this trend as the aftermath of the following:

> The distancing of religion from spirituality means that hospice workers are taught to believe that spirituality is about exploring personal meaning…. The concept of God is generally excluded …. The objective place of worship … in building hope and trust loses relevance. (Bradshaw, 1994, p. 416)

With this in mind, where is that relevance attached, if not the chapel? The answer was mentioned earlier: multi-faith rooms. The terminology here, as noted by Gilliat-Ray (2005), varies. Some of the terms used inter-changeably with 'multifaith rooms' are 'room of worship', 'prayer room' and 'quiet room'. I use the latter two terms in the next section, but not interchangeably. Unlike Gilliat-Ray (2005), I have found foundational dif-ferences between a prayer room and a quiet room, both in politics and the way the space is used.

The transformation of the 'sacred space'

Similar to images, until recently, small religious icons of Christian belief (i.e., small wooden crosses, small laminated icons of Jesus Christ) adorned the prayer/quiet rooms of the hospices. Following the trend of *casting off* religion, all such icons have now been removed from these spaces. Imperative is the following. *Prayer rooms* are renamed more and more into *quiet rooms*. This change may seem beneficial to some (moving away from religious language to promote neutrality), but to others this may cause dis-tress (lack of expression of focus on religious needs). To better explore this dichotomy, we should look at what the purpose of the prayer and quiet rooms has been.

Prayer rooms

Prayer rooms are designated spaces for people's prayers as well as peaceful places (Wright, 2001). The interior of the prayer room appears religious, but also is as a temple of spirituality (Hollins, 2006). Drawing on my project (Pentaris, 2016), religious symbols, like a crucifix, adorn the walls, a few CDs with prayers are placed on a small coffee table, the Bible, the Quran and some teachings of Hinduism in typed form are also on the table and available to whomever is making use of the prayer room.

No more than 10 months into the project, the prayer rooms were renamed *quiet rooms*. All quiet rooms were neutrally set up and, according to the clinical manager of one of the hospices, appropriate for all religious beliefs and none. What does a quiet room look like, though, as opposed to a prayer room? Walking in a quiet room, someone will now find a TV, DVD player, many DVDs and books, none of them relevant to religion or belief. Reminiscing Saunders (1988) words that hospice care should provide the individual with all the necessary resources for them to die peacefully, it seems that current politics and policy of hospice care find peaceful death in this new setting. The Bible was, in one of the wards, intentionally removed as 'it would have favoured Christians only and not be inclusive' (P.M., pers. comm., 13 June 2014). In addition to the DVDs and books, quiet rooms are equipped with board games and other family games.

In other words, quiet rooms resemble the neutral spaces in society, where religion and belief were, up until recently (also see Davie, 2013), not discussed or properly approached. Wilson (1966) argued that society secularises as it modernises. Similarly, one can argue that hospices are not primarily in the process of secularising. On the contrary, they are modernising and secularism comes with it hand in hand. This neutralisation of the sacred space is not a recent observation. Gilliat-Ray (2005) has explored extensively the transformation of the space from sacred to secular. Her observations derive predominantly from her research in prison chaplaincy but have a wider implication.

Quiet rooms

Hospice professionals and general staff members of a hospice are now also making use of a quiet room. To my experience, and drawing on Pentaris (2016) as well, healthcare professionals now either spend their break in a quiet room and have a nap, or have meetings about patients or take personal phone calls in the same space. During the course of my project (Pentaris, 2016), when interviewing professionals, often they would suggest that they have booked a room for our interview, and the room turned out to be the quiet room on the ward. This is the same experience as that of Pothoulaki, MacDonald and Flowers (2012); prayer rooms were booked to hold the interview sessions. This demonstrates the various ways in which these rooms are used nowadays. The rooms appear to be available for booking. Does that also suggest that patients and/or family members or friends who wish to make use of the space shall first make a booking?

It is indeed interesting to witness change in real time – from *prayer room* (i.e., a space provided for prayers and religious practise or practises associated with an individual's faith) to a *quiet room* (i.e., a room for personal insight and spiritual growth [K.F., pers. comm., 17 April 2014]) and, finally, even though it is still called a *quiet room*, to what seems to be a *recreation room*. These rooms are now equipped with all the appropriate material to amount to a recreation hall which offers activities (e.g., watching a film) that are far from keeping the space quiet in any way. I return to this point later in this chapter to link it with the use of hospice chapels and the gardens – a link which helps us progress our thinking about these spaces.

So far, in this section, we have seen how prayer rooms gave way to quiet rooms and, further, to the recreation use of the room. The transformation of the rooms, however, has preceded the realisation that they have transformed. If a quiet room is where an individual will go to find peace and explore their spiritual self (Wright, 2001), it is anticipated that a set of DVDs, a TV and a set of group games are defeating that purpose. On the contrary, the current neutrality from religion and belief increases the distance between the individual and their religious or non-identity; their need for spiritual care is sought to be met in a different space where particular identification of the person's religion and belief exists, or the individual has the freedom to initiate it. In other words, neutrality and impartiality in this space seems to be counterproductive as individuals may experience it as a subtle lack of identification of their identity and, therefore, the ability to exercise their faith in the hospice.

Finally, as quiet rooms appear to serve multiple purposes, what are the ethics for making use of them? When answering such questions, it is worth noting that different users have different purposes; it is no more a place of universal aim, but a hub that transforms based on the purpose it needs to serve each time.

Garden

Gardens are an integral part of a hospice building (McGann, 2013). The internal and external spaces have been designed to complement one another and, consequently, project a harmonious environment. McGann (2013, p. 93) appreciates how the garden may and should be placed in the centre of a hospice building: '[T]he garden completes the building space. Wrapping the building from around the garden space means that the garden then becomes the centre and focus of the building'.

Aside from how the hospice garden blends in to the remainder of the space, its purpose has seen some changes. In her work, McGann (2013) highlights that a garden is there to provide refuge, privacy and generally homely comforts. Drawing on Pentaris (2016), however, the garden has become a place for prayers and peacefulness; the space to accommodate whatever sacred was cast off from the prayer rooms. Icons and religious figurines are hidden in discreet places in the garden. During the time of my observations, I walked around the hospice gardens, looking for representations of religion and belief – religious icons or crosses or any signs that have been absent from the quiet rooms or the other spaces in the hospice. I was given the impression that I should be examining the garden, by patients and family members who have talked about the garden as the 'quiet place to be'.

Looking into the flower bushes and the pots with flowers, I spotted seven icons and four crucifixes in total. Religious images are placed inside the pots with the flowers (Figure 4.1), in places where a visitor would not think of. A couple of crucifixes were hanging from a thin string off the gazebo in one of the gardens and a rosary was hanging from a tree branch in another. All these items seemed to be carefully placed there whilst people would use the garden to pray or seek spiritual healing.

It is evident that the gardens have transformed conceptually into what Wright (2001) described as the functional role of a prayer room. Prayer rooms shall provide a peaceful place with the possibilities for religious practise, where the individual enjoys spiritual comfort. Regardless of its politics, and the way it is produced, as well as for whom (Gilliat-Ray, 2005), the findings of my study shed some light on the way that prayer rooms are used or not used (see 'Chapel' sub-section earlier in this chapter). Gilliat-Ray (2005) suggests a transformation of sacred spaces in public institutions, and her suggestions primarily include chapels and prayer rooms. What is found here

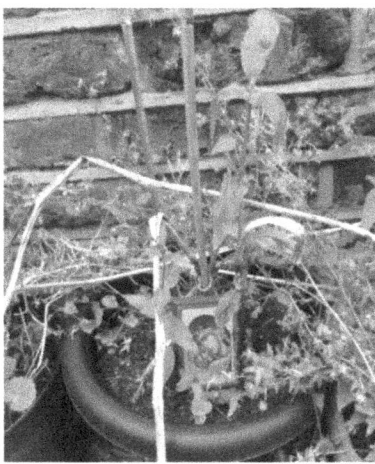

Figure 4.1 Retreating to the garden

Source: Photo by P. Pentaris

is that the sacred space keeps transforming and does not always remain the same physical space. From chapel to prayer room (Gilliat-Ray, 2005), from prayer room to quiet room, which then functions as a recreation room, and next to the garden (Figure 4.2).

Conceptually, the *sacred space* is something very personal and detached from institutionalised approaches. It is the space where an individual, religious or not, seeks to experience the sacred as personal, and express belief or disbelief about his/her experiences. However the identified need for spiritual care provision in EOL care, and in addition to the ongoing change of the name or title of the space used for related purposes, individuals seem to have felt needs (Bradshaw, 1972) which are yet to be met. The current arrangements in hospices (i.e., quiet rooms) appear not to address these needs and, therefore, individuals are using different spaces, such as the garden, where they have more freedom in action to seek spiritual comfort.

This is worrying, to an extent. If service users in hospices feel their needs are not met and seek alternative resources, even though policy has identified spiritual needs (Department of Health, 2009), there must be a gap in the communication between the two. Social policy (also see Chapter 3) seems to legislate guidelines that lack practise-based information, which makes for a challenging situation for all parties involved.

Figure 4.2 Transformation of the 'sacred space' in hospices

Case study

> *Maria's mother was in the hospice for a while to receive respite care. Maria felt overwhelmed with the care of her 92-year-old mother. She did not always find it easy to leave her mother at the hospice, especially as she felt there was not much time left for the two of them. When Maria dropped off her mother and the nurses made her comfortable in her room, Maria walked to the quiet room on the ward, where she found a medical professional and another staff member having a meeting. She was asked to return later, when the room would be available. As Maria wandered around the hospice – she wanted to make sure her mother was settled before she left – she found herself before the balcony door that led to the garden. There, she encountered a quiet corner bench in the garden. She sat down, took her rosary from her pocket, shut her eyes and started to pray.*

- *What did Maria need in that moment?*
- *What purpose does the garden play in this scenario?*
- *What are the ethics attached to use of the garden by Maria?*

This case study depicts one example of many in which individuals have sought not just privacy and refuge in the garden, but also a space where they can express their faith, religiosity or spirituality. Despite the difficulties in knowing all the ways people use to express their beliefs, my study draws on observations of people visibly praying, crossing their chest, kissing a religious icon and, very rarely (twice during my project [Pentaris, 2016]), sitting in a lotus position (i.e., cross-legged position in meditative practises).

Concluding thoughts

Spaces in hospices are visibly much more neutral over time. The experiences of secularisation that the public sphere has witnessed in the past 60 years are recently becoming evident in hospice care. The secularisation of EOL care might have started a lot more years before that (also see Walter, 2015); nevertheless, lack of social policy in the area, until a decade ago, as well as a lack of a healthy dialogue and communication among research, professional practise and social policy have led to the inability to identify how, what and why religion and belief are treated. The case of the transformation of the 'sacred space' is one of the examples that illustrates this.

During my study (Pentaris, 2016), I had the opportunity to discuss this information with ward managers, other staff members and members of the public, as well as patients. It is accurate that hospice managers, complying with organisational policies and procedures, discourage the use or presentation of any large religious icons in staff work areas, or religious icons in general on the wards. Although hospices respect professionals' wishes to wear a cross or have a small wooden cross attached to a frame on their desk, they request that all this be done discreetly and not at the expense of other people's beliefs or values. To do this, hospice policy recommends the avoidance of identification of the diversity one finds in these spaces, whilst it intentionally aims to promote neutrality and impartiality (also see Chapter 3). 'Things should be neutral and inclusive around here' said a staff nurse when asked during her night shift (J.O., pers. comm., 14 February 2014). Once again, this is evidence related to the debates around ideas of the secular (e.g., Wilson, 1966; Davie, 2015).

The idea of neutrality – when it comes to religion, belief and spirituality — seems almost impossible to me. Religion and belief are now recognised and protected characteristics in Equality Act 2010, yet the idea of neutrality recommends the opposite from identification. How could neutrality be sustained if religion was more visible, like race? For example, what if the conversation covered multi-ethnic environments and the intention was to be neutral and not show characteristics of hospice professionals' backgrounds to avoid exclusivity in hospice care? What if my ethnic background from Nigeria cannot *be* hidden when I am working with a white Irish service user? Would this indicate a lack of inclusivity? Would I be showing disrespect to the service user because my skin colour is different due to ethnic origin?

There is an uncanny belief that resides within professional practise, and often hospice professionals' mentality, that acceptance of one person's religion will result in biases against another's. On an organisational level, which then informs professional practise, there is the willingness of acceptance of people's social identities associated with religion and belief. However, there is seeming ambivalence towards acceptance.

Greer and Mor (1986) discuss how hospices, from social movement, became an institutionalised care for the dying, that later transformed into an institutionalised cure for the dying and the bereaved (Pentaris, 2014). The ambivalence for displaying a large religious icon on a hospice ward, for example, may be interpreted in a few different ways, not necessarily independent from each other. There is lack of religious literacy in relation to how space can be used by professionals when it has a religious character (i.e., there might be a need for integrating that reality into professional practise). Second, this is an additional sign of how hospices respond to Equality Act 2010, and especially the strand of religion and belief. There is poor understanding of hospice care, which stems from the organisational foundations and the core principles of the leadership teams – something that should be included in later studies.

Drawing from Hughes and Wearing's (2016) taxonomy of organisational theories, the hospice here may be considered either a cultural lens towards understanding EOL care further in general, or a living organism that sketches out the behavioural patterns within multi-professional environments. This chapter also reflects on the cultural dimensions of the hospice as an organisation. The way in which space is used is reflective of behavioural patterns within the system, and vice versa. The next three chapters put more emphasis on this claim and provide further information to support it.

References

Ammerman, N.T., 2016. Lived religion as an emerging field: An assessment of its contours and frontiers. *Nordic Journal of Religion and Society*, 9(2), pp. 83–99.

Bradshaw, A., 1994. *Lighting the lamp*. London, UK: Scutari Press.

Bradshaw, J., 1972. Taxonomy of social need. In: McLachlan, G. (ed.), *Problems and progress in medical care: Essays on current research, 7th series*. London, UK: Oxford University Press, pp. 71–82.

Bissell, G., 2012. *Organisational behaviour for social work*. Bristol, UK: Policy Press.

Cadge, W., 2013. *Paging God: Religion in the halls of medicine*. Chicago, IL: University of Chicago Press.

Cadge, W. and Konieczny, M.E., 2014. "Hidden in plain sight": The significance of religion and spirituality in secular organizations. *Sociology of Religion*, 75(4), pp. 551–563.

Csikai, E.L., 2006. Bereaved hospice caregivers' perceptions of the end-of-life care communication process and the involvement of health care professionals. *Journal of Palliative Medicine*, 9(6), pp. 1300–1309.

Davie, G., 2013. *The sociology of religion: A critical agenda*. London, UK: Sage.

Davie, G., 2015. *Religion in Britain: A persistent paradox*. Oxford, UK: Wiley-Blackwell.

Department of Health, 2014. *The mandate: A mandate from the government to NHS England: April 2014 to March 2015*. London, UK: Department of Health.

Department of Health, 2009. *Spiritual care at the end of life: A systematic review of the literature*. London, UK: Department of Health.

Evans, M.D., 2008. *Manual on the wearing of religious symbols in public areas*. Leiden: Brill.

Geertz, C., 1983. *Local knowledge*. New York, NY: Basic Books.

Gilliat-Ray, S., 2005. From 'chapel' to 'prayer room': The production, use, and politics of sacred space in public institutions. *Culture and Religion*, 6(2), pp. 287–308.

Greer, D.S. and Mor, V., 1986. An overview of national hospice study findings. *Journal of Clinical Epidemiology*, 39(1), pp. 5–7.

Hollins, S., 2006. Integrating spirituality in health and social care. *Nursing Management (Harrow)*, 13(3), pp. 6–7.

Horovitz, E.G., 2017. *Spiritual art therapy: An alternate path*. Springfield, IL: Charles C. Thomas.

Hospice UK, 2016. *Hospice care in the UK 2016*. London, UK: Hospice UK

Howard, E., 2013. *Law and the wearing of religious symbols: European bans on the wearing of religious symbols in education*. London, UK: Routledge.

Hughes, M. and Wearing, M. 2016. *Organisations and management in social work: Everyday action for change*. London, UK: Sage.

Insoll, T., 2009. Materiality, belief, ritual—Archaeology and material religion: An introduction. *Material Religion*, 5(3), pp. 260–264.

Johnson, R.L., Saha, S., Arbelaez, J.J., Beach, M.C. and Cooper, L.A., 2004. Racial and ethnic differences in patient perceptions of bias and cultural competence in health care. *Journal of General Internal Medicine*, 19(2), pp. 101–110.

Keane, W., 2008. The evidence of the senses and the materiality of religion. *Journal of the Royal Anthropological Institute*, 14(Suppl. 1), pp. 110–127.

Kellehear, A., Pugh, E. and Atter, L., 2009. Home away from home? A case study of bedside objects in a hospice. *International Journal of Palliative Nursing*, 15(3), pp. 148–152.

Mazzas, O., 2009. The right to wear headscarves and other religious symbols in French, Turkish, and American schools: How the government draws a veil on free expression of faith. *Journal of Catholic Legal Studies*, 48(2), pp. 303–344.

McGann, S., 2013. *The production of hospice space: Conceptualising the space of caring and dying*. London, UK: Routledge.

McGuire, M.B., 2008. *Lived religion: Spirituality and materiality in individuals' religious lives*. New York, NY: Oxford University Press.

Miller, D., 2005. *Materiality*. Durham, NC: Duke University Press.

Morgan, D., 1999. *Visual piety: A history and theory of popular religious images*. Berkeley: University of California Press.

Parkes, C.M., 1979. *Bereavement: Studies of grief in adult life*. London, UK: Routledge.

Pentaris, P., 2016. *Religious literacy in end of life care: Challenges and controversies*. Unpublished Doctoral Thesis (Goldsmiths, University of London).

Pentaris, P., 2014. Religion, secularism, and professional practice. *STUDIA Sociologica-Annales*, 6(1), pp. 99–109.

Pentaris, P., Papadatou, D., Jones, A. and Hosang, G., 2018. Professionals' perceptions on barriers and challenges when accessing children's hospice and palliative care services in the South East London: A preliminary study. *Death Studies*, 42(10), pp. 649–657.

Pothoulaki, M., MacDonald, R. and Flowers, P., 2012. An interpretative phenomenological analysis of an improvisational music therapy program for cancer patients. *Journal of Music Therapy*, 49(1), pp. 45–67.

Saunders, C., 1988. *St. Christopher's in celebration: Twenty-one years at Britain's First Modern Hospice*. London, UK: Hodder and Stoughton.

Stephenson, P.L., Draucker, C.B. and Martsolf, D.S., 2003. The experience of spirituality in the lives of hospice patients. *Journal of Hospice & Palliative Nursing*, 5(1), pp. 51–58.

Sue, D. W. and Sue, D., 2012. *Counseling the culturally diverse: Theory and practice*. Hoboken, NJ: Wiley.

Treviño, L.K., Butterfield, K.D. and McCabe, D.L., 1998. The ethical context in organizations: Influences on employee attitudes and behaviors. *Business Ethics Quarterly*, 8(3), pp. 447–476.

VandeCreek, L. and Burton, L. (eds.), 2001. Professional chaplaincy: Its role and importance in healthcare. *Journal of Pastoral Care & Counseling*, 55(1), pp. 81–97.

Vickers, L., 2016. *Religious freedom, religious discrimination and the workplace*. London: Bloomsbury Publishing.

Walker, A. and Breitsameter, C., 2017. The provision of spiritual care in hospices: A study in four hospices in North Rhine-Westphalia. *Journal of Religion and Health*, 56(6), pp. 2237–2250.

Walter, T., 2015. Secularisation. In: Parkes, C.M., Laungani, P. and Young, W. (eds.), *Death and bereavement across cultures* (2nd ed.). Abingdon, UK: Routledge, pp. 133–148.

Wilson, B.R., 1966. *Religion in secular society: A sociological comment*. London, UK: CA Watts.

Winslow, M. and Clark, D., 2005. *St. Joseph's Hospice, Hackney: A Century of Caring in the East End of London*. Brussels: Observatory Publications.

Wright, M.C., 2001. Chaplaincy in hospice and hospital: Findings from a survey in England and Wales. *Palliative Medicine*, 15(3), pp. 229–242.

Yancu, C.N., Farmer, D.F. and Leahman, D., 2010. Barriers to hospice use and palliative care services use by African American adults. *American Journal of Hospice and Palliative Medicine*, 27(4), pp. 248–253.

5 Hospice professionals and religion

Introduction

This chapter examines definitional issues between religion and spirituality as expressed by professional practitioners. It explores similarities and differences between their definitions and descriptions, taking into account general definitions of religion and belief as found in the sociology of religion. In addition, the chapter focusses on discussing hospice professionals' views about the following: first, how religion, belief and spirituality are linked with the experiences of dying and grieving, and second, how far service users' identities in these areas are important to their lives. More specifically, the chapter examines how hospice professionals appreciate the significance that service users may place in their religion, belief or spiritual identity in relation to their experiences of dying and grieving. This information provides an initial account of what may be expected in practise and highlights further educational needs or challenges that are then discussed in the last chapter of this book.

Separating religion from spirituality

Spirituality is an emerging area of research which lacks serious scientific history when addressed independently from religion (Egan et al., 2011. When religion is researched, spirituality tends to be embedded as a new religion or form of worship (Giordan and Pace, 2012). The challenge, then, is to overcome the tendency to use spirituality as a proxy when researching religion. The use of a proxy when studying religion is not a new theme, however; until very recently, the term 'culture' was used to refer to religion – an example being the edited collection *Death and Bereavement Across Cultures* by Parkes, Laungani and Young (2015). Their volume examines the various religious and nonreligious reflections on death and dying, but does so in the proviso that religion is culture and vice versa. This book, on the other hand, does not use any term as a proxy for another; rather, it examines the representation, expression, negotiation and management of religion, belief and spirituality in hospice care altogether. The term 'belief' is also inclusive of any set of beliefs which do not conform to religion or spirituality (e.g., nonreligion, secular beliefs).

Before we look at the views hospice professionals have about the role of religion in society and how they appreciate the importance that service users may attach to their beliefs, it is necessary to have a closer look at how professionals define and, therefore, understand religion and spirituality.

Defining religion and spirituality is a difficult task; both terms have various descriptions and meanings, and numerous scholars have offered their take on this matter. A most informative analysis of the definitions of the two terms is offered by Scott (1997). Scott was interested in how the terms 'religion' and 'spirituality' were understood in the 20th century. She examined 31 definitions of religion and 40 definitions of spirituality. Despite the similarities she identified in her analysis, her work is a perfect reminder of the complexity of these concepts; it highlights the inability of many 20th-century scholars to specify exactly what each of the terms means. Following this analysis, Zinnbauer, Pargament and Scott (1999) put more emphasis on the reality that there is no common definition of the terms and suggest that it is perhaps impossible to agree on one. The latter view is also seen in the work of Canda and Furman (2010), even though they do recommend a definition of spirituality in their work, and claim its wide applicability. Reflecting the view that no common definition can be agreed, Hill et al. (2000) asserted the following:

> Both spirituality and religion are complex phenomena, multidimensional in nature, and any single definition is likely to reflect a limited perspective or interest. In fact, it will be argued that past attempts to define these constructs are often too narrow, resulting in operational definitions that foster programs of empirical research with limited value, or too broad, resulting in a loss of distinctive characteristics of religion and spirituality. (Hill et al., 2000, p. 52)

Other scholars also stretch the uncertain definition of spirituality and seek benefits from it. Bregman (2004) argues that the vagueness of the term 'spirituality', or lack of a clear definition, should be seen as a positive sign as it allows professionals to shape and reshape the concept, dependent on the needs of their practise.

In general, religion has been characterised as an institution or a guided form of belief, whereas spirituality is seen as an individualised experience (Gall, Malette and Guirguis-Younger, 2011; Holloway and Moss, 2010). This separation of the two, however, as I have mentioned elsewhere (Pentaris, 2018), appears problematic. This is because for many people, religion is an individualised experience, or for others, their spirituality or spiritual practise may be organized (Pentaris, 2018). This is not a new argument but a reflection of Day's (2011) thesis of *believing without belonging* and *lived religion*; people may not belong to an institution but may still experience their religious belief on a more personal level.

As mentioned earlier, there are various definitions of the two terms available in literature and across various disciplinary areas. To benefit the purpose of this section (i.e., to examine how hospice professionals define and understand religion and spirituality), we first look at a few previous attempts to define the concepts of religion and spirituality. The latter will also help us make connections later with hospice professionals' descriptors of the same concepts.

Heelas (2002) considers religion to be God-centred – a view which reflects Pargament's (1999) conception of how religion turned from a 'broad-band construct' to a 'narrow-band construct'. Heelas appreciates religion as follows:

> '[R]eligion' has increasingly come to be seen as that which is institutionalized: involving prescribed rituals; established ways of believing; the 'official', as regulated and transmitted by religious authorities; that which is enshrined in tradition; the ethical commandments of sacred texts; the voice of the authority of the transcendent. (Heelas, 2002, p. 413)

One widely used definition of religion is that offered by Koenig (2009, p. 11): A system of beliefs and practises observed by a community, supported by rituals that acknowledge, worship, communicate with, or approach the Sacred, The Divine, God (in Western cultures), or Ultimate Truth, Reality, or nirvana (in Eastern cultures)'.

In contrast, definitions of spirituality put emphasis on meaning-making, expression of purpose and transcendence. An example is that of Puchalski et al. (2009, p. 887): 'The way individuals seek and express meaning and purpose and the way they experience their connectedness to the moment, to self, to others, to nature, and to the significant sacred'. Nevertheless, the concept of spirituality is not easily defined. This is best expressed by Crisp:

> It is perhaps not surprising that spirituality is not easily defined given that it is often concerned with intangible aspects of human life, with the capacity to move beyond that which is apparently rational. Furthermore, spirituality is a multifaceted concept. Hence attempts to define spirituality vary considerably as to what aspects are identified and prioritised by different writers. (Crisp, 2016, p. 10)

Equally, Hill et al. (2000) discussed the complexity of both phenomena: religion and spirituality. They identified spirituality as a multi-dimensional construct which needs be approached with great care. Some of the dimensions identified in spirituality are ultimate concern, yearning for meaning, integration with personality, identity and purpose, and connection with God. In general, Hill et al. (2000) argued that spirituality describes a personal experience whereas religion, despite its multi-faceted nature (i.e., social, personal and institutional), stipulates practises and traditions that guide the expression of belief. Roof (2003) draws on the disparities of religion and spirituality to attempt an integrated analysis of them, in which he proposes that they have a collaborative relationship. This reflects Schneiders' (2003) models of relationship between religion and spirituality, as well as James' (1961 [1902]) assertion that religion equates with spirituality, ignore institutional religion.

Schneiders (2003) discussed three models of relationship between religion and spirituality to reflect the way the concepts have been identified by scholars and the impact of such identifications. The first model proposes religion and spirituality as separate enterprises; the two are like "strangers" to each other with no connection. The next model proposes religion and spirituality as two conflicting realities 'related to each other in inverse proportion. The more spiritual one is the less religious, and vice versa' (Schneiders, 2003, p. 164). Finally, the third model that Schneiders described suggests that religion and spirituality are two dimensions of the same reality and are essential to each other. These models can be taken into account when exploring the various definitions and descriptors of these terms, to help us measure and understand the tensions between the meanings of the two terms.

Another conception of the terms has been proposed by Carrette and King (2005). These two scholars examined the way the term 'spirituality' has become popularised so widely and so quickly, at the expense of religion. They argue that spirituality, in western societies especially, can also be understood as a commodity (e.g., yoga, aromatherapy candles, meditative classes, ointments). In other words, the scholars perceived spirituality as a 'big business', representing a set of contemporary capitalist ideologies which have taken over religion and religious institutions.

The concepts of nonreligion, lack of religious affiliation and nonbelief are not necessarily addressed directly in this chapter, and it is worth explaining why that is. Zuckerman, Galen and Pasquale (2016) stress the value of nonreligion and secular beliefs, highlighting the moral responsibility to pay as much attention to these concepts as we do to the more conventional and substantiated ones. This study does not go into these concepts in detail, but takes as its starting point the most obvious binary (i.e., religion and spirituality) and attempts to tease out professionals' understandings of nonbelief (whatever the meaning) through their conceptions of belief. In other words, and drawing on Arweck, Bullivant and Lee's (2016) work, this book identifies the importance of these concepts, but accepts their relationship with religion and spirituality as described by hospice professionals.

In general, hospice professionals view religion as a constitution – a particular set of values that, when adapted, can shape and add value to an individual's experiences. In some senses, religion is presented as something that cannot be changed; religious beliefs are thought to be knowledge purely deriving from religious texts and teachings, and thus not subjectively perceived – indeed thought, on the contrary, to be measurable principles.

Despite the universal definitional characteristics of religion (i.e., a set of values and beliefs that acts as a guide in the believer's life) (also see Koenig, 2009), when intersected with spirituality its definition takes a radical shift and more intimate concepts (e.g., personal meaning) emerge. The study by Pentaris (2016), among hospice professionals, shows that religion is generally perceived as having a rigid and unchangeable character, but that when it is discussed alongside the concept of spirituality, it may become more open to questions. Drawing on Day's (2011) *believing in belonging* thesis and the dialogue around *cultural Christianity*, hospice professionals consider religion a form of culture or tradition, something inherited by people from older generations and traditionally followed or practised.

Religion

According to Pentaris (2016), hospice professionals define, describe or understand the term 'religion' in five different ways (Figure 5.1): guided lifestyle, set of beliefs, community, cultural system and source of knowledge.

Guided lifestyle

Professionals often appreciate religion as doctrine and understand its application either as following religious texts by the letter, or as the expression or acting out of religious teachings. In other words, hospice professionals frequently approach religion as a lifestyle characterised by rules and guidelines. This perception is not far from Kahoe's (1985) descriptions of mature religion (also see Allport and Ross, 1967). Kahoe (1985) explained functionally autonomous religion in two ways. First, he discussed intrinsic religion:

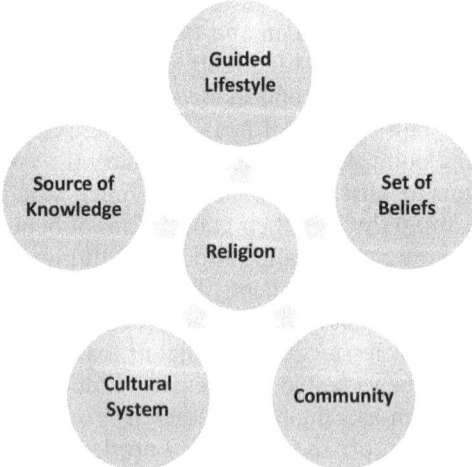

Figure 5.1 Hospice professionals' understanding of religion

an initially ego-centric view that progressed to include a more collective response to the world. In other words, intrinsic religion was connected to stereotypes and authoritarianism, but with little social applicability (Kahoe, 1977; Allport and Ross, 1967) as a result of its conservatism and perpetuation of superstitions. The second type of relationship between a person and their religion discussed by Kahoe (1985) was extrinsic religion. Once again, drawing on Allport and Ross (1967), Kahoe (1985) conceptualised the reasons for expressing religious texts through one's actions (i.e., extrinsic religion in simplistic terms).

Hospice professionals do not deviate from either of these two personal religious orientations (Allport and Ross, 1967), but perceive religion as a combination of all aspects of both. Although religious texts are appreciated as sets of rules and guidelines which inform a person's self, professionals also view a person's actions as representative and as inextricably linked with their belief.

Set of beliefs

As well as observing Johnstone's (2015) sociological appreciations of religion and Bowen's (2017) approach to the anthropology of religion, hospice professionals also view religion as an organised set of beliefs which have been passed down through generations, either by tradition or by teaching. Drawing on Pentaris (2016), professionals have often highlighted that religion is not just about belief; rather, people are taught rituals and practises that define a religion and help them understand it as a set of such beliefs. This idea is widely represented in Woodhead, Partridge and Kawanami's (2016) work about the transformative character of religious traditions in the modern world. In their edited volume, a number of scholars are invited to discuss various religions within the confines of traditional practises – an attempt which further supports the connections hospice professionals make between tradition and belief.

Community

Religious communities have often been explored in terms of resources. For example, Koenig (2009) and Robinson and Hanmer (2014) examined the importance of religious communities in the informal support systems of people and the establishment of robust approaches to prevent child abuse and neglect. Equally, religion and religious belief have been explored in relation to chronic illnesses and imminent death. The consensus is described in Jenkins and Pargament (1995): Both religion and spirituality are perceived as key resources which can help patients, family and friends cope with an illness and its progression.

Thus, hospice professionals often identify religion as a community and support system. As one hospice professional phrased it: "It is like the centre of the town. We come together as a community because of religion". In addition, professionals appear to show appreciation of religion as a resource for support. Service users often require extensive support, which might come from informal and voluntary arrangements, including their religious community and its leaders.

Cultural system

Other professionals in hospices were less assertive about their understanding of religion. It was recognised as a form of culture with historical elements, but little evidence is available to support whether hospice professionals who appreciate religion as culture also have the insight to tell the two things apart. Such insight would suggest a more robust perspective.

Source of knowledge

Hospice professionals with more than 20 years of experience in end of life care suggest more broadly that religion is a source of knowledge. Often, hospice care has a medical basis whereas religious belief provides answers to questions that medicine and clinical practise cannot – namely, existential questions pertaining to the end of one's life (Tomer, Eliason and Wong, 2013; Feifel, 1959). Thus, hospice professionals with longer experience in the field negotiate their understanding of religion and its role based on the purpose it serves; *it offers answers when no one else can.*

Spirituality

On the other hand, spirituality is presented as a subjective experience, not dissimilar to what other researchers and authors have found elsewhere, as described earlier in this chapter. Hospice professionals refer to spirituality with the descriptions of meaning, identity and personal interpretations – all reminiscent of Ricoeur's (1976) interpretation theory – otherwise known as 'the theory of language'. Ricoeur established hermeneutics as a field, as well as a method of study to discuss the ways in which messages, texts, discourses and so on are interpreted. Equally, spirituality becomes an experience subjected to interpretation, both by the self and the other.

'Spirituality' is a complicated term that lacks definition, mainly due to disagreement among researchers and theorists (also see Lazaridou and Pentaris, 2016). The need to define the term, or at least address it in this way here, is that we come across it in social policy and health regulations concerning holistic approaches and person-centred care. What hospice professionals offer in Pentaris (2016) is a clear understanding that spirituality is something personal and it refers purely to the meaning individuals develop about their life as it passes (Figure 5.2).

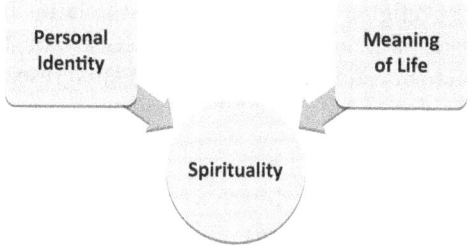

Figure 5.2 Hospice professionals' understanding of spirituality

Personal identity

More rarely, but reminiscent of Gebelt and Leak's (2009) work about the interrelationship of spirituality and identity, hospice professionals considered spirituality a form of identity or an indication of one's personal identity. The emphasis here is placed on the person's history, personal values, experience, lifestyle, and general character. Namely, the conception presents itself as inclusive of any background and is based on the proviso that all individuals are spiritual, regardless of whether they acknowledge it, whether they consider themselves religious or nonreligious and whether they adhere to the beliefs of atheism or agnosticism. This is not my own argument, and it is not a new one.

Starting from Nee's work (1998), the idea of *the spiritual man* has been promoted by various scholars. Nee delves into a journey in which he examines a procedural experience of spirituality, with the proviso that all people are spiritual. Nee goes on to recommend that because people are either misguided or not guided at all, they are often unable to express their spiritual identity. Thus, Nee's recommendation that all individuals are spiritual is reflected in hospice professionals' views and in the ways that professionals separate religion and spirituality.

Meaning of life

By and large, hospice professionals, not unlike those in other areas of practise (Hill and Pargament, 2008), approach spirituality as transcendence. The predominant understanding of spirituality here is that it highlights what gives meaning to the individual. It is understood as a concept which expresses not only how people find meaning in their lives, but also the extent to which they find a place and purpose. Broadly, hospice professionals perceive this term as one that explains a person's beliefs, religious or not, whereas they recognise spirituality as something larger than religion – beyond doctrine, or traditional or conventional practises.

The way hospice professionals perceive, understand and explain spirituality is critical to how spiritual beliefs are integrated in practise. In fact, the differentiation of religion and spirituality – the latter including nonreligious, atheist, secular and agnostic beliefs – sets a robust platform upon which we can further (beyond this book's arguments) research the place of religion and belief in end of life care more broadly.

The role of religion in society

In Chapter 2 we were reminded of the contemporary challenges of religion in society. The concepts of secularism, post-secular communities and religious institutions all have a part to play in this (also see Davie, 2015) and are reflected in professionals' views. The previous section put emphasis on professionals' appreciation of religion, spirituality and consequently other orientations of belief (e.g., secular ideas, atheism, non-secularity). With this in mind, this section reports on how hospice professionals appreciate the role of religion, and faith more generally in society.

When exploring how professionals in hospices understand and embed religion, belief and spirituality in their practise, it is just as important to gather insight about what their thoughts are in relation to religion's place in society in general. Professional literature across disciplines, personal values, opinions and attitudes – research-informed or not – all play key parts in the professional's practise (Hamberger and Moore, 1997). Equally, conceptions and misconceptions are important as we tend to project them in our everyday lives (Goffman, 1999).

Figure 5.3 lists professionals' conceptions of religion's role in society as they emerge from Pentaris (2016). Broadly, professionals in this area appear to think of religion's place in society in four main ways (among others which are discussed later): that religion has lost its significance in society; that rather than being a tradition or embedded cultural identity that is passed down through generations, religion is a choice; that religion provides a

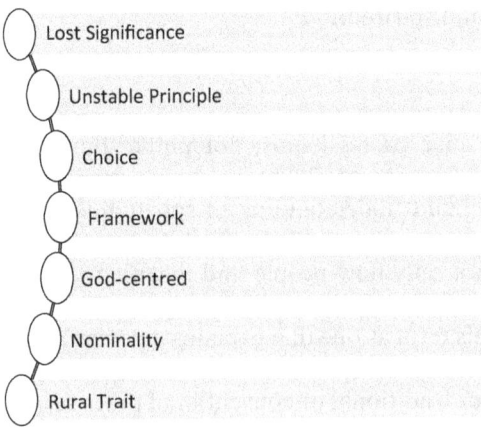

Figure 5.3 Hospice professionals' perceptions of religion in society

framework which informs the way people wish to be cared for and that religion is an unstable principle.

Lost significance

Famous sociologist Brian Wilson attested in the 1960s (Wilson, 1964) that religion is heading towards a place where it will lose its social significance. He examined societal changes through the lens of modernity, yet did not account for the significance of religion within individual consciousness. Many theorists and scholars followed Wilson's thesis and examined secularity and post-secularism extensively, yet only in the past 20 years have we seen the dialogue progressing towards the idea that religion and belief did not lose social significance, but rather that society is experiencing shifting ways of expressing belief and its relation to its functions.

By and large, these views appear to have naturalised in hospice care. Approximately 50% of the hospice professionals who took part in my study (Pentaris, 2016) stated confidently that religion is no longer as important in society and that people no longer perceive or appreciate religion in the same as they did in the past. This is not far from Carrette and King's (2005) argument that spirituality 'took over' religion and became a way of discussing religion as well as other themes such as transcendence, individuality and compassion.

Hospice professionals also appear to perceive religion as something that is not important in society, extending this view to conclude that it is also not as significant to individuals. Such stances may suggest, however, that religion and belief are both poorly regarded in professional practise. Some examples of this position are seen in Box 5.1.

Religion is considered an insignificant matter in society, and thus professionals show less interest in engaging in the conversation. For example, to return to the points made earlier in this section, the debates from early

---

Box 5.1

'I mean … you hear the statistics, which you do not know, and they quote like two-thirds of the population are unsure of their religion, or are agnostic or atheist and only a third are actually practising some form of religion; somewhat fifty thousand are … This is us – Jedi minds or whatever. So, I mean, you get the impression that, in society in general, religion seems to be having less of an importance' (John, age 53).

'Well, you know, people are not really religious, are they? I guess it is not that important and … well it depends I guess' (Janice, age 47).

'[N]ot very important, is it? I mean, everybody says that religion is declining and all, you know. Even the chaplain here says so, so I guess … well, it does not seem that people think that it is important anymore …?' (Nick, age 41).

sociologists (e.g., Wilson, 1966) suggest that religion has been steadily losing significance in society. Nonetheless, numerous scholars, including Dinham (2015), Davie (1994, 2007), and Hervieu-Léger (2000), argue that religion, religious belief and religious practise have not been lost from the public sphere, but have rather changed their nature. Hospice professionals are not unwilling to engage with this strand of social identity; however, lack of public recognition and conversation about religion and belief leads to a lack of courage in engaging with the subject within hospice care. I return to this argument in Chapter 8.

During my fieldwork, the following was rather informative of the material just covered. When discussing 'religion' with professionals, the conversation naturally shifts towards creeds, whereas when the concept of 'belief' is specified, the conversation flows in a different direction, becoming more 'spiritual'. This further supports the claim that professionals shy away from talking about religion, whereas discussing spirituality, belief and meaning-making makes for a more comfortable conversation. However, it is yet not evident, due to a lack of data, whether these perceptions of what is and is not important in professional practise are informed by service user worldviews as well (see Beresford, 2000).

Perceptions of lost significance, or any of the following categories, become important indicators of how religion, belief, and spiritual identities are perceived and integrated into hospice professionals' appreciation of an individual's experiences, influencing professional practise. This is also illustrated by the following: Parkes, Laungani and Young (2015) reviewed different religious groups and their responses to the experiences of death, dying and bereavement. The review was based on the principle that religious belief is a significant aspect of an individual's understanding of his or her experiences. The study on which this book reports (Pentaris, 2016) adds that these are issues which do have an impact on professional practise in hospices.

Unstable and unnecessary principle

Another perception we find in hospice professionals' thoughts is that religion is regarded as an institution that has 'fallen apart'. Leaving aside the perceived value of particular guidance by religious leaders, the core principles and values of religion are seen as unstable and even unorthodox at times (Box 5.2). Other professionals may go beyond 'unstable' characterisations and talk about religion as an *unnecessary social identity*.

If, however, hospice professionals do not consider religion and belief as necessary, despite their being perceived as so by dying and/or bereaved individuals (Pentaris, 2011; De Hennezel, 2007; Leming and Dickinson, 2010; Parkes, Laungani and Young, 2015), a large gap between service users' needs, service provision and service delivery arises. Lack of acknowledgement of needs related to religion and belief, or lack of the right language to address them, may lead to inadequate services.

Box 5.2

'Religion used to have to offer something, hope.... it is unfortunate ... it does not anymore ... it feels like something unstable these days and it is sad ... people find it unstable' (Jeremiah, age 58).

'It feels like something that has let loose, and it feels very unstable and those are things that are falling apart [in society]' (John, age 53).

'It has turned into something very unstable. You believe and you do not believe; it is the same thing. So, religion is not necessary' (Alex, age 44).

Finally, if religion is considered an unnecessary and unstable principle, this is exacerbated by the absence of religion and belief from the physical space (see Chapter 4) – the removal of religious artefacts from hospices mirroring hospice professionals' declining view of its stability.

Religion as choice

In Sartre's work (2016 [1948]) about existentialism and humanism, we come across the power of will and choice. Sartre argued that in life we make a choice to follow one system of belief over another and that, even if we later become dissatisfied by that choice, we were still given the option initially. Similarly, professionals may also consider belief and religion a choice; we choose to believe or not believe (Box 5.3).

Professional attitudes towards understanding and perceiving religion and belief are paramount to professional practise (also see Pentaris, 2014). If religion is indeed a choice, should that choice not be the individual service user's to make? This perception brings about various challenges; the most

Box 5.3

'Historically, religion was more like a thing. It was not a choice. Now it is more of a choice' (Carol, age 42).

'You are raised with values. Whether you frame them with religious beliefs that is a choice you have in life' (Nick, age 41).

'Well, it is not something that people have to do. You can choose not to believe, can you not?' (Jenny, age 24).

'Religion is just something that we choose to do. I guess there is no one to tell you when and how. You know, you will decide if you want to go to Sunday Church or not' (Shahid, age 33).

'Religion might had been important in the past, but now it is just a choice. There is nothing else to it, is there?' (Margarita, age 36).

'It is not really something that interests me anyways, but I just say that it is one of the choices in life' (Raul, age 26).

obvious is that if religion or belief is a choice, do we also agree that believing in or affiliating with one religion over another is the product of the capacity to make a choice? Where does this perception leave individuals who may lack such capacity (e.g., those with mental health problems)? What about children and belief? Does this perception suggest that a five-year-old child, unable in his or her primary developmental stage to make an informed choice about religion or belief, cannot be religious by nature? Such questions are not answered here, but I find this conversation rather galvanising towards future research.

Religion as a framework

Religion is further described by hospice professionals as a framework which dictates or is used to interpret how religious people experience their lives. Interestingly, participants in my study (Pentaris, 2016) approached this description in two different ways. A few hospice professionals suggested that religion is of great importance in society as it provides a framework that people use to guide their lives. However, many others described religion as guidelines and frameworks as only of importance in directing an individual's life, if chosen.

This theme also emerges in policy documents (e.g., End of Life Care Strategy 2008 [Department of Health, 2008]; also see Chapter 3). How religion and belief are addressed in hospice care truly reflects how religion has been conceptualised as a framework with particular guidelines and specificities that direct a person's experiences. For example, the latest brief on the NHS Improving Quality document (Department of Health, 2013) suggests that it is important to have prayer mats in institutions when Muslim patients are admitted.

This example also raises a challenge and poses a question which is addressed later in this chapter. Do hospice professionals base their professional practise on the assumption of religious belief which stems from religious affiliation? Furthermore, if religion and belief are a set of rules that create a 'path' for people to follow through life, then this should be where professionals involved in the delivery of EOL care (characterised by empathetic and person-centred approaches) meet dying or bereaved individuals and families. The discussion becomes more complicated if we also consider debates about secularity and secular professional practise.

Religion as realisation of The Divine

An additional perception recorded in hospice professionals' thoughts is that the role of religion in society is to enable individuals to come to terms with the knowledge of a god, any god. Religion, here, is described as the proof of realisation of The Divine – a proof that individuals are aware of something larger than themselves (Box 5.4).

Box 5.4

'It is people having an awareness, any awareness, that religion, any religion, that there is a god, that we are not the most important things, and it is having respect for a being above us who puts us here' (Gita, age 59).

'Whether you go to the synagogue, the mosque, or wherever you go, make sure you take time out and go and thank that God and show respect to somebody that is bigger and better than me, that I do not fully understand, and be thankful for what we have' (Janice, age 47).

The realisation of The Divine is not merely an idea of what God is, but a stance: a personal attitude towards religion and belief. This may have a two-fold implication to how hospice professionals incorporate the realisation of The Divine in their professional practise. On the one hand, acknowledging the importance of someone's belief system and religious identity has to them shows respect and comprehension. However, this attitude raises the expectations of service users. Thus, this stance works exclusively regarding nonreligious people, or people that are of a religion by tradition and not by belief.

In addition, views about religion and belief in society might also indicate personal beliefs. Some professionals identify God as the authority and see prayer and obedience as an obligation of the believer or follower. But where does this leave service users who are aware of the reality of a higher power but do not subscribe to these obligations? Does this stance create more barriers than bridges in communication between professionals and service users? After all, religious literacy is also about having the language to communicate openly about religion and belief without expressing a strong believing in one thing over the other (Pentaris, 2018).

Religion as nominal statement

Some professionals consider religion to be something insignificant, but nonetheless important to include in their description of themselves. Such position is neither insignificant nor foreign to scholarly work from the 1960s and more recently.

In his work, the American cultural anthropologist Spiro (1966) examined nominal definitions of religion. 'Nominal definitions are those in which a word, whose meaning is unknown or unclear, is defined in terms of some expression whose meaning is already known' (Spiro, 1966, p. 85). In other words, a nominal perception of religion would indicate that the person expressing it understands or appreciates the meaning and role of religion based on the expressions surrounding it.

Similarly, reminiscent of Day's (2011) suggestions on performative religion, people often claim a religious identity or affiliation as it results from

---

Box 5.5

'Someone can say I am Church of England as a nominal statement' (Raul, age 26).
  'Sometimes you say Christian because that is what your family is, or even say I guess I am Jewish Orthodox, because that is how you have grown up' (Margarita, age 36).

---

culture and tradition. The meaning of religious identity, then, is the product of cultural engagement with that identity.

Drawing on both Spiro's (1966) and Day's (2011) work, hospice professionals appear to express expectations of a culturally bound response to the question: What is your religion? Some extracts from research findings are presented in Box 5.5 to illustrate this point.

Day (2009), in her ethnography of young people, argues that religion is connected with power and authority and that it suggests links with socially constructed religious belief. Later, Day and Lynch (2013) proposed different ways in which religion and belief are experienced as cultural performances. Performing belief due to cultural background is a nominal statement (also see Voas and Crockett, 2005). Similarly, hospice professionals' attitudes towards religion and belief resemble a performance, or at least a performative experience (Day, 2011).

That said, there is a higher risk of false assumption in professional practise. If the religious identity of service users is understood as cultural identity with no significant aspects of belief and meaning-making in life, professionals may oversee how the individual perceives his or her aspect of religion and belief. If so, the risk of unmet needs in hospice care is higher and the quality of care is put in question.

Lived religion in rural areas

An additional theme worth exploring is the perception that religion is treated differently in rural areas as opposed to urban ones. Vidich and Bensman (1968) explored the different functions of various aspects of a small community in New York in the 1960s, including looking at what religion meant to the community. Specifically, in their monograph, they suggested that Sunday mornings were solely dedicated to churchgoing, when all members of the community would dress in their best outfit and attend church. The situation described by Vidich and Bensman is not dissimilar to more recent examples. For example, Poliakov and Olcott (2016) explore the Islamic tradition and lived faith in rural communities in Asia.

Drawing on the current research, hospice professionals who live in rural areas present themselves with different perceptions of religion and its role in society. This knowledge highlights that quality of care is also informed by the residency or origins of professionals. This is not to suggest that being from a rural area indicates higher levels of quality of care, or the opposite. However, it is an important aspect of reality which contests the ideology of care.

Religion, belief, spirituality and dying

This section continues to explore hospice professionals' views about the relationship between religion and death, but puts emphasis on how those perceptions play out in practise.

Garces-Foley (2014) examined the various challenges in this discussion and highlighted the dearth of information about how religion and death intersect in a social context. It is this aspect, rather than the rites and practises assigned to dying and grieving by different religions, that interests me the most (also see Davies, 2017). In other words, this book discusses how hospice professionals understand and appreciate the complementary relationship between death and religion on a social level to explore the functions of religion for those experiencing the loss of a loved one, or for those dying themselves.

The findings from Pentaris (2016) demonstrate a general understanding that religion acts as a facilitator towards gaining better familiarity with an imminent death or a recent loss by death. Although this understanding leads us to think that religious text/beliefs/rites dictate the meaning of the forthcoming experience (i.e., death), it goes beyond that (or needs to). In particular, human experience is a social construct dependent on personal, relational and societal values, and subject to criticism; in these terms, religion adds to the social construction of the experience of dying and grieving.

In Pentaris (2016), it appears that hospice professionals attest to four ways in which religion relates to death, dying and bereavement (Figure 5.4). The following sections discuss all four categories.

Nonreligion and dying

Nonreligion is a fast-growing field of study which only recently took ownership of its terminology (Lee, 2012). Nonetheless, nonreligion as an

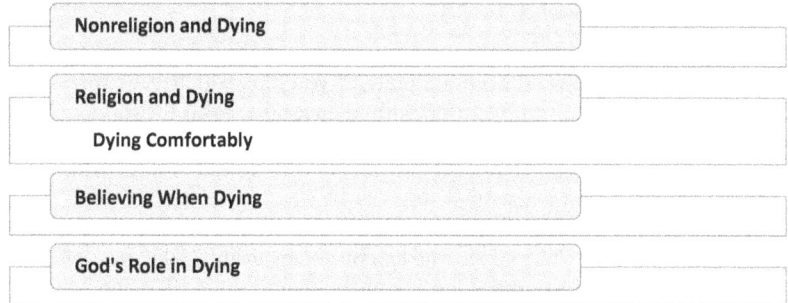

Nonreligion and Dying

Religion and Dying

Dying Comfortably

Believing When Dying

God's Role in Dying

Figure 5.4 How does religion relate to death, dying and bereavement?

identity has been negated or nullified (LeDrew, 2013), further distorting public opinion of its legitimacy. In relation to death, dying and bereavement, nonreligion is as important a view as any other. However, it is evident from my research that hospice professionals differentiate their views about service users' experiences based on whether they identify as nonreligious or religious.

We already know that religion or religious belief is significant when making sense of the experiences of death, dying and bereavement (Garces-Foley, 2014). We also know that belief, religious or not, is imperative to how one experiences death and grief (Pentaris, 2011). However, my study (Pentaris, 2016) shows that hospice professionals' views may vary, and often suggests that lack of religious belief results in ignorance when approaching the end of life or the experience of grieving (Box 5.6). Drawing on Garces-Foley (2006), the perception that nonreligious service users are simply unaware of their experience and unable to find meaning in them is questionable. Garces-Foley (2006) examined the politics of spirituality within hospice care in the US and highlighted both the negative association of religion and external doctrines, and the positive associations between spirituality and the yearning for truth and meaning. What is questionable about the perception discussed in this sub-section is not whether it is true, but rather the underpinning thought which led to this perception. If we take Garces-Foley's (2006) work into account, it seems to me that hospice professionals examine religion as an internal process of search for meaning, while equating nonreligious with nonspiritual and considering nonspiritual somehow lacking.

Borrowing from Feifel's work (1977, p. 6), it is important to be reminded here that 'death is for all seasons'. If belief is a season, then death is for all beliefs. Belief is not always religious and death is not always direct. All these factors are notable in the consideration of whether nonreligious individuals are 'ignorant'. Nonetheless, we are still in an era of end of life care, in which 'dying and death are now the province of the "professional"' (Feifel 1977, p. 5). Therefore, it is still significant to address professional practise and/or social policy deficiencies and/or adequacies.

Box 5.6

'There is a drive to try and accommodate, if you like, whichever expression of faith or religion is given by an individual encounter with the family. And you know, even for people who are a bit more lost and have no means to make sense of what is going on, you know like people with no faith or agnostics, we do the same' (Margarita, age 36).

'People without faith are probably happier when they are dying, as they are ignorant about the afterlife and have no fear of … judgement' (Johannes, age 39).

'Some patients will say that God is not for them, but if they appreciated that the end is near, they would be less ignorant' (Johannes, age 39).

It appears that there is the tendency, within hospices, to use 'ignorance' and 'nonreligion' as interchangeable and interconnected terms. This raises many challenges and questions concerning professional practise, and how current thinking of nonbelief in society plays out in this sector. Becker (1973) suggests there is always belief in something and that this is precisely what motivates people. Moreover, philosophy (e.g., Ricoeur, 2008) suggests that ignorance may be the guide of lacking something about something else. What is argued in this book is that the lack of religious literacy may lead hospice professionals to have flawed perceptions of the ways in which religion, belief and spirituality are perceived and experienced by service users.

In addition, this thought brings more challenges, which may be covert. One such challenge is the following: Professional practise benefits from the service user's religious belief. To explain further, religious teachings give answers. There are answers in relation to dying, death, the afterlife and judgement or purification. These are answers far from the scientific, clinical and bio-medical approaches of hospice care, and therefore not handled by physicians or nurses. In the event that a dying individual does not have a religious belief, there is also the possibility that the answers about what happens next have not been given. What if the individual then turns to medical, clinical and allied staff for answers? Do hospice professionals feel uncomfortable in addressing these issues due to lack of non-scientific status, leading to a perception of nonreligion as ignorance in dying? Of course, this is merely a speculation, but with legitimate grounds for further research in the area.

Religion and dying

Various scholars (e.g., Kastenbaum, 2015; Pentaris, 2011; Argyle and Beit-Hallahmi, 2014) have explored the possibility that religious belief enhances the experience of death. Kastenbaum (2015) further explored the multi-dimensional ways in which the experience is enhanced, not simply on a personal level, but also on societal and political levels. Equally, Pentaris (2016) highlights that hospice professionals perceive religion and belief in general to be significant elements in how service users experience death, dying and bereavement (Box 5.7).

Box 5.7

'If we can relate to death in a meaningful way, that would be religion and spirituality. We sort of have to involve our spirituality, I think, to be able to deal with death or accept death in a healthy way' (Shahid, age 33).

'I think the link between the two is when people are looking for meaning for their life. So, if people are religious, it means that they have a God, they hope that they have done their best for their God in this earth in life, and then they will go onto heaven, or where Allah is taking them, or where Jewish believe they will go' (Mirna, age 48).

Religious and/or spiritual belief (whatever the meaning) may enhance the experience of death by providing meaning in life.

An alternative view of how religion enhances the experience of death is through symbolism. Being mindful of post-Kantian theories of symbolism that stress the need for a distinct separation between symbols and signs, as well as drawing on the philosophical and conceptual analysis of symbols and language by Urban (2014), we ought to approach this view with great care. Symbols are not simply signs which indicate one thing over another; rather, it is the meaningful nature of a sign which turns it into a symbol, a form of communication conveying what is important or insignificant for an individual.

Along similar lines, professional practise within hospices recognises that it is not necessarily religion as doctrine or a belief system which enhances the experiences of death, dying and bereavement, but religious symbols and icons, and the importance service users attach to them. This is yet another contradictory conception, if we look back at hospice mandates requiring hospice spaces to remain neutral from religion to facilitate inclusivity. This contrast is further discussed in Chapter 8.

The theme of 'enhancement', coupled with that of 'ignorance', introduces a wider argument about the levels of religious literacy of hospice care. Specifically, we find hospice professionals who suggest that 'nonreligion' equals *ignorance* whereas 'religion' equals *enhancement*. In other words, people with nonreligious beliefs would not enjoy enhanced experiences of dying and bereavement. How comfortably can we accept this, however, and how does hospice care today work towards tackling the questions arising from this information? In other words, is hospice care designed and delivered on the foundation of such stereotypes or misconceptions?

Dying comfortably

It is conspicuous in previous literature (Davies, 2017; Pentaris, 2016; Garces-Foley, 2014) that hospice professionals appreciate that religious beliefs, as well as spiritual, lead to a comfortable and peaceful death for the individual. Dying is a crisis in itself. The idea of a deteriorating body and numerous future losses might be hard to cope with, but religion makes people feel comfortable. Equally, the expression of grief comes with crises. Religion may provide comfort to the bereaved – family members and friends who are seeking to understand and accept the event of death.

Reming and Dickinson (2005) review the ways in which people find comfort and peace in their dying or other people's dying. The dying process has been described as a lonely one (De Hennezel, 2007; Elias, 1985). Levine (1989) stresses that the individual can experience a conscious death as the result of a preceding conscious life. If the latter is missing, dying becomes an uncomfortable experience, similar to a lived discomfort looking into the unknown. Religion and belief are important aspects of the enhancement of the experience, and the alleviation of some of the anxieties accompanying death, as well as the means towards a conscious life and death. A recent source of literature that reflects on this is by Parkes et al. (2015).

Believing when dying

This category is, not exclusively, based on Elias' (1985) thoughts on *the loneliness of the dying*. It is suggested that individuals experience their own dying in a lonely environment even if they are not alone. Close to the end of their lives, people show more openness in the religious/spiritual aspects of their identity; and thus, signs of belief are stronger. Hospice professionals who contributed to Pentaris' study (2016) suggested that patients are prone to believing (whether that refers to a particular religion or any belief) when death is imminent and its inevitability is ascertained (Box 5.8).

According to Saunders (2005), patients who are close to the end of life, tend to experience a spiritual quest (also see McSherry and Ross, 2010) and find themselves challenged by the irreversible and inevitable reality of an end' to opportunities for future experiences, reflections and/or doing right or wrong. Life as they know it comes to an end (Feifel, 1959). What patients at this stage are left with, according to Field (2002), is the uncertainty of the when, how and why. The findings from Pentaris (2016) show that hospice care considers religion and belief to be the answer to these questions.

Kellehear (2000) describes three sources of meaning amounting to a theoretical model of spiritual needs. He identifies three blocks of spiritual building in palliative care: the situational, the moral and biographical, and the religious. The situational, here, refers to the dying state and the context within which dying is taking place. The ethical and biographical highlights the moral history of the individual – what the principles and values that have been passed on to them by tradition or culture contribute to the individual's spirituality in dying. Last, the religious refers to religion and belief. Similar to Kamath's (1978) philosophy of dying, religion is the most ancient medicine for the dying and the bereaved. Religious practise and death rituals are what link the deceased's departure with the grief of the living.

This argument may appear to contradict previous research findings indicating that the older the person, the more religious they are

---

Box 5.8

'If they are facing the fact that they are dying, their life comes towards an end, that can sometimes make them focus on their spirituality or religion in a way that they might not have done previously' (Alex, age 44).

'I think as people get closer to death, in many cases, they look at their own mortality, and perhaps speak an expression of a kind of religion. They [dying persons] may start seeking what they have not before, like meaning and life after death' (Dorothy, age 37).

(also see Blazer and Palmore, 1976; Levin, 1998). However, the following is important to note: The current argument does not contest the relationship between ageing and religion. On the contrary, it often places this relationship within the context of a hospice.

Davie and Vincent (1998, p. 101) explored what surveys had indicated regarding older people and religion/belief, and suggest that 'older people ... have always been more religious than the young'. Research literature (Levin, 1998) and sociological explorations (Phillips, Ajrouch and Hillcoat-Nallétamby, 2010) largely support this. Simultaneously, studies have never rejected the idea that death interrelates with religion (Garces-Foley, 2014). In this book, I reflect on research findings from Pentaris (2016), in which hospice professionals share views that expect religious needs to increase as service users' draw nearer to the end of their lives. However, the findings do not show from what experiences professionals are drawing this view.

According to my project (Pentaris, 2016), hospice professionals identify that the connection between death, dying and bereavement, and religion is created at the time of dying, if not earlier. In general, there seems not to be an expectation that established religion and belief may precede this point, but that religion and belief are either established in that moment in life (i.e., dying or grieving) or are magnified when the individual gets nearer to the experience. The question for both social policy and professional practise, therefore, is: During their initial admission, should service users be asked, if religious, how much their belief has magnified since the change in their health circumstances?

God's role in dying

Often, also noted by De Hennezel (2007), hospice professionals perceive that religion or religious teachings and beliefs impose judgement and eventually punishment on the individual (Box 5.9). It is discernible from Pentaris (2016) that hospice professionals, alongside their perception that dying individuals become more religious, tend to appreciate an adverse perspective of religion when it comes to linking it with illness and death, dying and bereavement experiences.

Drawing on both this category (God's role in dying) and the previous (believing when dying), a contradiction arises: religion, belief, spirituality,

---

Box 5.9

'You have people who are very devout and sometimes they see it as a form of punishment. Or: 'Why is this happening to me?', 'Have I done anything wrong?', 'Do I deserve this?' (Janice, age 47).

'People feel anger and disappointment towards God. Fair enough people have the right to feel distressed and angry, particularly if they are young and they are losing young children' (Anna, age 59).

nonreligion and any other faith seem to be described, in hospice care, as actors of either punishment or reinforcement, or both. This is an ambiguous contrast which requires analysis on its own. Punishment for whom and by whom? Reinforcement by whom, for whom and to whom? Such questions need further research and analysis, but from a multidisciplinary approach, to capture more fully the complexities of these concepts and current professional responses to religion, belief and spiritual identities in hospice care.

The role of religion, belief and spirituality for service users

There is a general understanding that service users attach significant meaning to their religious beliefs (Parkes et al., 2015). Even if individuals have not been religious throughout the course of their lives, when death approaches they tend to reminisce about and rediscover their religious beliefs and seek comfort from them (Garces-Foley, 2014). Ardelt and Koenig (2006) examined the negative and positive correlations between intrinsic and extrinsic religious orientation, and the experiences of older hospice patients. In their findings, they highlighted that older hospice patients seem to find meaning in or through their religion and/or belief as well as seek comfort in the answers religion provides, that are not compatible with scientific methods.

This section, however, does not review current literature regarding what the functions of religion and belief are for service users in hospice care. Rather, it highlights current views and attitudes by hospice professionals about the matter to situate better the following chapter, as well as the overall arguments of this book.

In general, hospice professionals show a lack of understanding concerning religion and belief's importance to service users. To explain further, hospice care is built on the premise of empathy and person-centred practise; so, one would expect it to recommend perfect appreciation of individual experiences. To the contrary, according Pentaris (2016), hospice professionals largely – but not exclusively – appeared uncertain and unclear about the functional roles of religion, belief and spirituality to the service user's experience. Beyond this challenge, five categories emerged, which illustrate how hospice professionals comprehend the role of religion and belief for service users (Table 5.1).

Meaning-making

Despite the different opinions regarding what the role of religion and belief is, as well as the disparities between what is considered religion and what is spirituality, the majority of hospice professionals find that religion and belief often assist in meaning-making. This is not a new finding, but it emphasises how professionals appreciate, and therefore connect with, service users' religious beliefs and spiritual identities.

Table 5.1 The role of religion and belief for service users

Category	Description
Meaning-making	Religion and belief assist in making meaning in life events such as death, dying and bereavement.
Cultural beliefs	Religion and belief are mere traditions of the family or society/country of origin of the individual.
Universal spirituality	There is no individual without spirituality or religion.
Unique understanding of religion and belief	Religion and belief are individually understood concepts.
Decision-making	Religion and belief assist in making significant decisions in life.

Furthermore, Newton and McIntosh (2013) explored extensively the contributions of religion in meaning-making processes. An extraordinary finding of their analysis is that religion and religious belief make meaning more meaningful. Specifically, religion acts as an interpreter of human experience, signifying the way meaning is understood. If we completely accept this analysis, however, are we to accept that the meaning that nonreligious people make is less meaningful than others?

Evidently, according to this study, hospice professionals agree that spirituality, religious or not, has inner and existential purposes (Box 5.10). Individuals seek making sense of their experiences, and spirituality is an important way in which they do so.

In addition to meaning-making, hospice professionals consider religion and belief to assist towards reflective meaning-making – in other words, to reflect on what service users' accomplishments in life have been and how their life events have led them to where they are at the time of their death or grieving. If service users find such immense comfort and meaning in religion and belief, then hospice care has a responsibility to provide services which adequately and appropriately respond to such needs, and to avoid the risk of inclusivity and equity in care being counterproductive to this responsibility (Pentaris, 2018).

Box 5.10

'I think, for some people, their religious part of their lives is phenomenally important and they want that to be recognised, and it is quite important to their identity and to their meaning; how they make sense' (Cirik, age 46).

'People have to make sense of what is happening to them in the context of their understanding of the world and their understanding of religion. It is a big part from what I have witnessed' (Margarita, age 36).

Cultural beliefs

Requests or wishes expressed by service users are often interpreted as beliefs that stem purely from tradition and not from within the individual's consciousness. This directly links to Day's (2011) thesis of performative religion and cultural Christians. Similarly, hospice professionals who contributed to this study discussed *cultural Jews, cultural Muslims* and others.

Furthermore, it is not uncommon for hospice professionals to equate religious practises with cultural practises (e.g., Kelley and Morrison, 2015). Nonetheless, these are said to be respected and well-received in terms of advance directives and within the context of holistic hospice care (Sprung et al., 2014).

In the face of future changes in hospice and palliative care (Etkind et al., 2017), explicit policy seems to be lacking. Policy should not only address conceptual needs on a theoretical basis, but also be presented in the right language to professional practise. Equally important, policy for hospice and palliative care should show thorough understanding of the difference between accommodation of requests and the integration of faith, belief or values, and principles.

Universal spirituality

Service users are seen as spiritual beings, often tantamount to religious (Box 5.11). The challenge with this is twofold. First, this statement contradicts the idea that spirituality is a very personal matter and can only be defined as such. With this in mind, the category *universal spirituality* seems provocative. Second, spiritual care has been embedded in hospices as the means to respond to religious needs. Therefore, there is the question of whether nonreligious people are seen as religious in hospices and, if so, why and what for?

Unique understanding of religion and belief

Along the same lines of considering religion and belief as important aspects of an individual's identity, hospice professionals in general suggest that the

---

Box 5.11

'I think people are not necessarily aware … you know, of their spirituality. It [spirituality] is there and it is alive but they [people] are not aware of it, sort of still living through them but not able to explain it or they might not think that they are spiritual' (Mary, age 29).

'In my experience, everybody has a spiritual identity. I think it is incredibly rare not to have a spiritual identity' (Shahid, age 33).

'I do not think I have met a person who is not at least spiritual' (Michael, age 43).

'Spirituality is very important. People, no matter what their religion is or not or whatever, they are spiritual' (Alex, age 44).

122 Negotiating belief in hospice care

level or type of importance the individual ascribes to religion or belief is completely aligned with their personal association with it. Once again, we often come across literature (e.g., Parkes et al., 2015) which associates religion with culture, whilst emphasising the individualistic interpretation of people's faith (also see Day, 2011) as well as contextual meaning-making through experiences of death, dying and bereavement.

Decision-making

Kwak and Haley (2005) are but one example of many who examine the role of religion in decision-making in end of life care. They reviewed a wide range of research findings to identify the various ways in which religion is relevant to end of life decision-making among ethnically diverse populations. Religion and belief appear to play an important part in end of life decision-making and this is explored further in this book.

This argument is imperative given the principles of person-centred care. Lack of religious literacy may lead to lack of understanding of the service users' decisions, which may affect treatment, pain management or other agreements, such as advance directives. This is a significant challenge that appears to contribute to religion and belief's lack of integration into professional practise, as we see in the next chapter.

References

Allport, G.W. and Ross, J.M., 1967. Personal religious orientation and prejudice. *Journal of Personality and Social Psychology*, 5(4), pp. 432–443.

Ardelt, M. and Koenig, C.S., 2006. The role of religion for hospice patients and relatively healthy older adults. *Research on Aging*, 28(2), pp. 184–215.

Argyle, M. and Beit-Hallahmi, B., 2014. *The psychology of religious behaviour, belief and experience*. New York, NY: Routledge.

Arweck, E., Bullivant, S. and Lee, L. (eds.), 2016. *Secularity and non-religion*. London, UK: Routledge.

Becker, E., 1973. *The denial of death*. New York, NY: Free Press.

Beresford, P., 2000. Service users' knowledges and social work theory: Conflict or collaboration? *The British Journal of Social Work*, 30(4), pp. 489–503.

Blazer, D. and Palmore, E., 1976. Religion and aging in a longitudinal panel. *The Gerontologist*, 16(1), pp. 82–85.

Bowen, J.R., 2017. *Religions in practice: An approach to the anthropology of religion*. London, UK: Routledge.

Bregman, L., 2004. Defining spirituality: Multiple uses and murky meanings of an incredibly popular term. *The Journal of Pastoral Care and Counselling*, 58(3), pp. 157–167.

Canda, E.R. and Furman, L.D., 2010. *Spiritual diversity in social work practice: The heart of helping*. Oxford, UK: Oxford University Press.

Carrette, J.R. and King, R., 2005. *Selling spirituality: The silent takeover of religion*. London, UK: Psychology Press.

Crisp, B.R., 2016. *Spirituality and social work*. London, UK: Routledge.

Davie, G., 2015. *Religion in Britain: A persistent paradox*. Oxford, UK: Wiley-Blackwell.

Davie, G., 2007. Vicarious religion: A methodological challenge. In Ammerman, N.T. (ed.), *Everyday religion: Observing modern religious lives*. New York, NY: Oxford University Press, pp. 21–36.

Davie, G. and Vincent, J., 1998. Religion and old age. *Ageing & Society*, 18(1), pp. 101–110.

Davies, D., 2017. *Death, ritual and belief: The rhetoric of funerary rites*. London, UK: Bloomsbury Publishing.

Day, A., 2011. *Believing in belonging: Belief and social identity in the modern world*. Oxford, UK: Oxford University Press.

Day, A., 2009. Believing in belonging: An ethnography of young people's constructions of belief. *Culture and Religion*, 10(3), pp. 263–278.

Day, A. and Lynch, G., 2013. Introduction: Belief as cultural performance. *Journal of Contemporary Religion*, 28(2), pp. 199–206.

De Hennezel, M., 2007. *Ο μύχιος θάνατος: Οι ετοιμοθάνατοι μας μαθαίνουν τη ζωή [The intimate death: The dying teach us life]*, Athens, Greece: KOAN/Synergie.

Department of Health, 2013. *NHS Improving Quality*. London, UK: Department of Health.

Department of Health, 2008. *End of life care strategy: Promoting high quality care for all adults at the end of life*. London, UK: Department of Health.

Dinham, A., 2015. Religious literacy and welfare. In Dinham, A. and Francis, M. (eds.), *Religious literacy in policy and practice*. Bristol, UK: Policy Press, pp. 101–112.

Egan, R., MacLeod, R., Jaye, C., McGee, R., Baxter, J. and Herbison, P., 2011. What is spirituality? Evidence from a New Zealand hospice study. *Mortality*, 16(4), pp. 307–324.

Elias, N., 1985. *The loneliness of the dying*. New York, NY: Blackwell.

Etkind, S.N., Bone, A.E., Gomes, B., Lovell, N., Evans, C.J., Higginson, I.J. and Murtagh, F.E.M., 2017. How many people will need palliative care in 2040? Past trends, future projections and implications for services. *BMC Medicine*, 15(1), pp. 1–10.

Feifel, H., 1977. *New meaning of death*. New York, NY: McGraw-Hill.

Feifel, H. (ed.), 1959. *The meaning of death*. New York, NY: McGraw-Hill.

Field, D., 2002. Preparation for palliative care: Teaching about death, dying and bereavement in UK medical schools 2000-2001. *Medical Education*, 36(6), pp. 561–567.

Gall, T.L., Malette, J. and Guirguis-Younger, M., 2011. Spirituality and religiousness: A diversity of definitions. *Journal of Spirituality in Mental Health*, 13(3), pp. 158–181.

Garces-Foley, K., 2014. *Death and religion in a changing world*. London, UK: Routledge.

Garces-Foley, K., 2006. Hospice and the politics of spirituality. *Omega: Journal of Death and Dying*, 53(1), pp. 117–136.

Gebelt, J.L. and Leak, G.K., 2009. Identity and spirituality: Conceptual and empirical progress. *Identity: An International Journal of Theory and Research*, 9(3), pp. 180–182.

Giordan, G. and Pace, E., 2012. *Mapping religion and spirituality in a postsecular world*. Leiden: Brill.

Goffman, I., 1999. *The presentation of self in everyday life*. Gloucester, MA: Peter Smith.

Hamberger, N.M. and Moore Jr, R.L., 1997. From personal to professional values: Conversations about conflicts. *Journal of Teacher Education*, 48(4), pp. 301–310.

Heelas, P., 2002. The spiritual revolution: From 'religion' to 'spirituality'. In Woodhead, L., Fletcher, P., Kawanami, H. and Smith, D., (eds.), *Religions in the modern world*. London, UK: Routledge, pp. 417–436.

Hervieu-Léger, D., 2000. *Religion as a chain of memory*. New Brunswick, NJ: Rutgers University Press.

Hill, P.C. and Pargament, K.I., 2008. Advances in the conceptualization and measurement of religion and spirituality: Implications for physical and mental health research. *Psychology of Religion and Spirituality*, 58(1), pp. 3–17.

Hill, P.C., Pargament, K.I., Hood, R.W., McCullough Jr, M.E., Swyers, J.P., Larson, D.B. and Zinnbauer, B.J., 2000. Conceptualizing religion and spirituality: Points of commonality, points of departure. *Journal for the Theory of Social Behaviour*, 30(1), pp. 51–77.

Holloway, M. and Moss, B., 2010. *Spirituality and social work*. Basingstoke, UK: Macmillan International.

James, W., 1961. *The varieties of religious experience: A study in human nature*. Cambridge, MA: Harvard University Press. (Original work published 1902).

Jenkins, R.A. and Pargament, K.I., 1995. Religion and spirituality as resources for coping with cancer. *Journal of Psychosocial Oncology*, 13(1–2), pp. 51–74.

Johnstone, R.L., 2015. *Religion in society: A sociology of religion*. London, UK: Routledge.

Kahoe, R.D., 1985. The development of intrinsic and extrinsic religious orientations. *Journal for the Scientific Study of Religion*, 24(4), pp. 408–412.

Kahoe, R.D., 1977. Intrinsic religion and authoritarianism: A differentiated relationship. *Journal for the Scientific Study of Religion*, 16(2), pp. 179–182.

Kamath, M.V., 1978. *Philosophy of death and dying*. Honesdale, PA: Himalayan Institute.

Kastenbaum, R., 2015. *Death, society and human experience*. London, UK: Routledge.

Kellehear, A., 2000. Experiences near death: Beyond medicine and religion. Brisbane, Australia: Replica Books.

Kelley, A.S. and Morrison, R.S., 2015. Palliative care for the seriously ill. *New England Journal of Medicine*, 373(8), pp. 747–755.

Koenig, H.G., 2009. *Faith and mental health: Religious resources for healing*. West Conshohocken, PA: Templeton Foundation Press.

Kwak, J. and Haley, W.E., 2005. Current research findings on end-of-life decision making among racially or ethnically diverse groups. *The Gerontologist*, 45(5), pp. 634–641.

Lazaridou, A. and Pentaris, P., 2016. Mindfulness and spirituality: Therapeutic perspectives. *Person-Centered & Experiential Psychotherapies*, 15(3), pp. 235–244.

LeDrew, S., 2013. Discovering atheism: Heterogeneity in trajectories to atheists' identity and activism. *Sociology of Religion*, 74(4), pp. 431–453.

Lee, L., 2012. Research note: Talking about a revolution: Terminology for the new field of non-religion studies. *Journal of Contemporary Religion*, 27(1), pp. 129–139.

Levin, J.S., 1998. Religious research in gerontology, 1980–1994: A systematic review. *Journal of Religious Gerontology*, 10(3), pp. 3–31.

Levine, S., 1989. *Who dies? An investigation of conscious living and conscious dying*. New York, NY: Bantam Doubleday Dell Publishing Group.

McSherry, W. and Ross, L. (eds.), 2010. *Spiritual assessment in healthcare practice*. London, UK: M&K Update.

Nee, W., 1998. *The spiritual man*. Anaheim, CA: Living Stream Ministry.

Newton, T. and McIntosh, D.N., 2013. Unique contributions of religion to meaning. In Hicks, J.A. and Routledge, C. (eds.), *The experience of meaning in life: Classical perspectives, emerging themes, and controversies*. New York, NY: Springer, pp. 257–269.

Pargament, K.I., 1999. The psychology of religion and spirituality? Yes and no. *The International Journal for the Psychology of Religion*, 9(1), pp. 3–16.

Parkes, C.M., Laungani, P. and Young, W. (eds.), 2015. *Death and bereavement across cultures*. London, UK: Routledge.

Pentaris, P., 2018. The marginalization of religion in end of life care: Signs of microaggression? *International Journal of Human Rights in Healthcare*, 11(2), pp. 116–128.

Pentaris, P., 2016. *Religious literacy in end of life care: Challenges and controversies*. Unpublished Doctoral Thesis (Goldsmiths, University of London).

Pentaris, P., 2014. Religion, secularism, and professional practice. *STUDIA Sociologica-Annales*, 6(1), pp. 99–109.

Pentaris, P., 2011. Culture and death: A multicultural perspective. *Hawaii Pacific Journal of Social Work Practice*, 4(1), pp. 45–84.

Phillips, J.E., Ajrouch, K.J. and Hillcoat-Nallétamby, S., 2010. *Key concepts in social gerontology*. London, UK: Sage.

Poliakov, S.P. and Olcott, M.B., 2016. *Everyday Islam: Religion and tradition in rural Central Asia*. London, UK: Routledge.

Puchalski, C., Ferrell, B., Virani, R., Otis-Green, S., Baird, P., Bull, J., Chochinov, H., Handzo, G., Nelson-Becker, H., Prince-Paul, M. and Pugliese, K., 2009. Improving the quality of spiritual care as a dimension of palliative care: The report of the Consensus Conference. *Journal of Palliative Medicine*, 12(10), pp. 885–904.

Leming, M.R. and Dickinson, G.E., 2010. *Understanding dying, death, and bereavement*. Andover, UK: Cengage Learning.

Ricoeur, P., 2008. *Freud and philosophy: An essay on interpretation*. Delhi, India: Motilal Banarsidass Publishe.

Ricoeur, P., 1976. *Interpretation theory: Discourse and the surplus of meaning*. Fort Worth, TX: TCU Press.

Robinson, M. and Hanmer, S., 2014. Engaging religious communities to protect children from abuse, neglect, and exploitation: Partnerships require analysis of religious virtues and harms. *Child Abuse & Neglect*, 38(4), pp. 600–611.

Roof, W.C., 2003. Religion and spirituality. In Dillon, M. (ed.), *Handbook of the sociology of religion*. Cambridge: Cambridge University Press, pp. 137–148.

Sartre, J.P., 2016 [1948]. Existentialism and humanism (1947). In Baggini, J. (ed.), *Philosophy: Key texts*. London, UK: Springer, pp. 115–133.

Saunders, D.C., 2005. *Cicely Saunders – Founder of the Hospice Movement: Selected letters 1959-1999*. Oxford, UK: Oxford University Press.

Schneiders, S.M., 2003. Religion vs. spirituality: A contemporary conundrum. *Spiritus: A Journal of Christian Spirituality*, 3(2), pp. 163–185.

Scott, A.B., 1997. *Categorizing definitions of religion and spirituality in the psychological literature: A content analytic approach*. Unpublished manuscript.

Spiro, M.E., 1966. Religion: Problems of definition and explanation. In Banton, M. (ed.), *Anthropological approaches to the study of religion*. London, UK: Association of Social Anthropologists of the Commonwealth, pp. 85–96.

Sprung, C.L., Truog, R.D., Curtis, J.R., Joynt, G.M., Baras, M., Michalsen, A., Briegel, J., Kesecioglu, J., Efferen, L., De Robertis, E., Bulpa, P., Metnitz, P., Patil, N., Hawryluck, L., Manthous, C., Moreno, R., Leonard, S., Hill, N.S., Wennberg,

E., McDermid, R.C., Mikstacki, A., Mularski, R.A., Hartog, C.S. and Avidan, A., 2014. Seeking worldwide professional consensus on the principles of end-of-life care for the critically ill: The consensus for Worldwide End-of-Life Practice for Patients in Intensive Care Units (WELPICUS) study. *American Journal of Respiratory and Critical Care Medicine*, 190(8), pp. 855–866.

Tomer, A., Eliason, G.T. and Wong, P.T. (eds.)., 2013. *Existential and spiritual issues in death attitudes*. Hove, UK: Psychology Press.

Urban, W.M., 2014. *Language and reality: The philosophy of language and the principles of symbolism*, vol. 69. London, UK: Routledge.

Vidich, A.J. and Bensman, J., 1968. *Small town in mass society: Class, power, and religion in a rural community*, vol. 131. Champaign, IL: University of Illinois Press.

Voas, D. and Crockett, A., 2005. Religion in Britain: Neither believing nor belonging. *Sociology*, 39(1), pp. 11–28.

Wilson, B., 1966. *Religion in secular society*. London, UK: C.A. Watts.

Woodhead, L., Partridge, C. and Kawanami, H. (eds.), 2016. *Religions in the modern world: Traditions and transformations*. London, UK: Routledge.

Zinnbauer, B.J., Pargament, K.I. and Scott, A.B., 1999. The emerging meanings of religiousness and spirituality: Problems and prospects. *Journal of Personality*, 67(6), pp. 889–919.

Zuckerman, P., Galen, L.W. and Pasquale, F.L., 2016. *The nonreligious: Understanding secular people and societies*. Oxford, UK: Oxford University Press.

6 Hospice professionals and religious literacy

Introduction

The previous chapters have made clear the leading challenge with measuring religious literacy: It is a fluid, context- and person-specific concept. Thus, it is difficult for any researcher to be certain when a professional is religious literate and at what level. However, by means of observation and follow-up discussions, and with appropriate methodologies, it is not impossible to record professionals' knowledge, skills and ability to engage with religion, belief and spirituality.

This chapter describes hospice professionals' knowledge and understanding of and skill and ability to respond to religion-, belief- and spiritual-related needs of the dying and/or bereaved. The chapter examines the interplay between professionals' willingness to engage with care on this level and their ability to do so. It does so by means of case studies, providing readers with in-depth understanding.

In detail, the chapter examines the depth and breadth of knowledge about religion, belief and spirituality indicated by hospice professionals' views. Drawing on other literature and my research (Pentaris, 2016), this chapter explores two main areas: hospice professionals' views about knowledge exchange in hospice care (which increases skills and abilities in practise) and professional limitations and lack of understanding of religion and belief when providing care to people for whom religion, belief and spirituality are important. Specifically, the chapter discusses practically how hospice professionals respond practically to service user needs related to religion, belief and spirituality.

Knowledge and understanding of religion and belief

Following on from the concept of religious literacy (Dinham and Francis, 2015), it is only appropriate that we explore not only the knowledge of religion, belief and spirituality that hospice professionals acquire in the field, but also their understanding of it as well as their willingness to expand on it.

Figure 6.1 depicts how hospice professionals appreciate their knowledge and understanding of religion and belief. This figure shows that

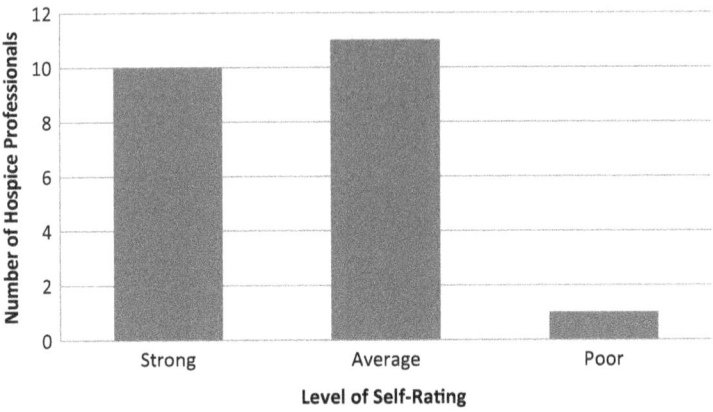

Figure 6.1 Self-rated knowledge and understanding of religion and belief

approximately half of the professionals who participated in Pentaris' (2016) study considered themselves to have a strong knowledge background of religion and belief and a good understanding of it, whereas the other half (approximately) recognised room for improvement. This information suggests various scenarios, perhaps some being assumptions due to be researched.

Many hospice professionals appear to approach the question of how much knowledge and understanding they have about religion and belief from a Christian-centred perspective (Pentaris, 2016). This finding is not uncommon. In various previous works (e.g., Li, 2004), professionals approached the subject through a lens of superiority – from a dominant perspective. Sociology has long studied dominant and non-dominant groups in societies; a powerful analysis of such work has been done by Knowles and Peng (2005). They examined the concept of 'white' as an ethnic identity. In their analysis, they highlighted the default dominance of the identity and how that impacts societally on various levels. Of course, there are political, social, historical, environmental and economic reasons for certain groups becoming dominant in society. Christianity, for example, has predominated in the UK for over 1,500 years. This historical fact, and the way various forms of Christianity have naturalised and embedded in the public morality and environment, means it is inevitable that members of this society experience life through a Christian lens.

Despite the change in the way hospice professionals respond to religious needs, if a Christian lens applies, the following is also challenging. It is often evident, in my research experience, that when researching religion or belief, research participants tend to separate the dominant religious denomination from other religions, traditions or spiritualities. This leads to the assumption that research is focussing primarily on how professional practise deals with religions other than the dominant, which causes uncertainty from a theoretical and research perspective. This is where cultural humility also becomes relevant (Hook et al., 2003). Aside from respect for the other, cultural humility is also concerned with a lack of superiority – in other words, addressing the other from an equal perspective and not through the lens of dominance. In addition, when hospice professionals consider faith as something primarily religious, where does that leave people of no faith, spiritual or not?

The argument of the superiority with which hospice professionals address religion, belief and spirituality supports London's (2008) review comments that Anglican churchmen relied on their pre-existing Christian-centred worldview to address new issues. Similarly, hospice professionals appear to evaluate their level of engagement with religion, belief and spiritual identity based on their Christian-centred knowledge and understanding (of course, this suggestion should be generalised with caution, given the mixed background of hospice professionals themselves [also see Kronenfeld, 2010]).

To appreciate better hospice professionals' knowledge about religion and belief, I separate the various in the following sections to present the conceptions and contestations in this area.

Knowledge about religion and belief

Acquiring new knowledge, as well as sustaining and/or developing current knowledge, are principal ideas in hospice care. Professionals appear committed to these ideals and are willing to engage with as many training and educational opportunities as necessary to expand or explore their knowledge about religion and belief. However, and this is one of this book's arguments, willingness to commit to such activities is dependent on the person's self-awareness about the need to enhance or gain new knowledge. In other words, this section of the chapter seeks to present to what extent professionals consider their knowledge developed or developing and by what means it could be developed.

Knowledge by assumption

British philosopher Alfred Jules Ayer dedicated his career to the pursuit of an understanding of knowledge and truth in the context of logic. His work *The Problem of Knowledge* (Ayer and Marić, 1956) is one of the most comprehensive, but contested, examinations of knowledge and its logic. Ayer breaks free from the conventional ways of perceiving knowledge and accepts true belief as knowledge, as long as certain circumstances apply. In other words, Ayer questions the distinction between knowledge and true belief, and asserts: 'For it is possible to be completely sure of something which is in fact true, but yet not to know it' (Ayer and Marić, 1956, p. 29).

Very simple examples can highlight the quote just presented. For instance, one may be completely sure that it will rain, but not know it. In a similar vein, hospice professionals present themselves as having abundant true belief, but not necessarily knowledge about it. In Ayer and Marić's (1956) words, this may not be problematic, but what appears to be is the belief that the true belief *is* knowledge. On the other hand, Ayer and Marić (1956, p. 32) also recommend that 'normally we do not say that people know things unless they have followed one of the accredited routes to knowledge'. Therefore, making assumptions can be argued as part of a routine path towards accrediting knowledge. This, however, is not of concern to this book.

Drawing from my study (Pentaris, 2016), it seems that many hospice professionals assume their knowledge and understanding of religion and belief, as well as assume the factors that will get them engaged with these parts of the identities of service users. It is apparent that professionals, on the one hand, argue about their comfort and set of skills to engage with religion, belief and spiritual identities. However, when asked directly about these issues, there is a hesitancy in responding clearly.

When professionals were asked about knowledge and understanding of religion and belief (Pentaris, 2016), and how practise integrates such identities, they used vocabulary such as 'think', 'probably', 'might', 'guess', 'would suggest', 'possibly know' and 'assume'. The choice of words indicates uncertainty of knowledge. It suggests the respondents may have not been challenged to answer these questions before and therefore indicates a lack of thorough analysis of how, when and why such social aspects of individuals' identities can be integrated in practise.

Linking the discussion about a Christian-centred lens in practise with the origins of the hospice movement (Saunders, 2005) is unavoidable, as is the inevitable link with professionals' confidence in their knowledge. The care of the dying and the bereaved in the West has historically been driven by Christians and delivered in a Christian-centred context. Inevitably, the principles and values of hospice care developed around Christianity, and thus similar principles became central to the education of professionals in the hospice sector, and in healthcare more generally. Nonetheless, the ongoing changes in the composition of the population – cultural and religious diversity – demand further competency building and training. This has generally been taken into consideration. However, how such emerging needs in education and training have been looked at reflects a Christian lens and a secular-minded approach (also see Davie's 2015 review *Religion in Britain*).

One of the most controversial issues here is how one claims knowledge about a concept about which one lacks understanding, such as nonreligion or atheism. Only a small amount of research (e.g., Smith-Stoner, 2007) has focused on nonreligious or atheist hospice patients, and even less work is available to shed light on whether hospice professionals understand these unique identities. It became evident from my study that hospice professionals assumed each patient and their families to be spiritual, regardless of religion or the lack of it, and therefore made the assumption that every person needs spiritual support.

There are two ways of looking at this. First, as systemic oppression (Feagin, 2013): Lack of appreciation of the potential that current practises or mindsets could be oppressive toward individuals is a very serious concern. I have recently examined a similar concern (Pentaris, 2018), in my study about the impact of lack of religious literacy in end of life care. I argue that instances such as this may result in microinvalidations which often have a hurtful outcome for the patients, their families and friends. The second way in which we can appreciate the assumption that everyone is spiritual relates to Ayer and Marić's (1956) work on the problem of knowledge. Ayer asserts that a true belief (other known as a 'guess') can turn into knowledge if 'proved' true repeatedly. However, some key questions arise from this: When does a series of successful assumptions become knowledge? At what and to whose expense? To whose benefit?

Once again, there is an element of assuming knowledge. An additional and important suggestion (although made with caution), is that there is a tendency to cluster religious and nonreligious people as 'nice' and 'not nice' people, respectively. Drawing on Pentaris (2016), it was not rare for hospice professionals, in their attempt to come across as open and comfortable with all different forms of faith, to betray their discomfort by suggesting that nonreligious people 'can be nice as well', even when the question has not been intended to address this matter.

The latter partly links to Campbell's work (1977). In it, Campbell argues that *irreligion* is an important aspect of religion, and refers to the acts and processes of rejecting religion. When nonreligious service users are perceived as 'not nice', the following argument is raised: Are the hospice professionals who suggest this religious? And this is, perhaps, a type of judgemental attitude which jeopardises the service delivery in the long run? Or is this pure coincidence, and when hospice professionals say that nonreligious people are also nice, they are showing their use of this coping mechanism that allows them to *understand* something different from what they *believe*? No matter which is true, the present book shows that hospice professionals need to acquire adequate knowledge and understanding about religion and belief.

Basic knowledge

Questions regarding the knowledge and understanding of religion and belief aim to address how professionals in hospices, and in end of life care more generally, respond to the diverse faith identities they come across in practise. Scholars on the subject include the following: Daaleman and VandeCreek (2000) suggested that religion and belief have not yet found their appropriate place in EOL care. Hermann (2000) found that dying patients have unmet needs around the spiritual aspect of their identity, regardless of whether it includes religion. O'Connor (1988), in the late 1980s, suggested that professionals have not yet acquired the full skillset needed to meet spiritual needs of service users.

There is a general acceptance of mainstream knowledge, attained mainly through professionals' own religious background (e.g., professionals claimed to have acquired knowledge about various religions because they are Christians themselves). Also, hospice professionals present themselves as open to identifying their education, or lack thereof, as a barrier which may limit their knowledge in this area.

It is clear in Pentaris (2016), however, that we may be facing conceptual misunderstandings of faith. Professionals, especially those with extensive experience in end of life care, recommend that having some basic knowledge of different religions (e.g., times of prayers per day for Muslims) amounts to proper religious literacy and effective professional practise in hospice care. These indications have similarities with O'Connor's (1988) group of professionals, who also claimed basic knowledge of religion. Such indicators can also be examined through the lens of my recent work on religious microaggressions in end of life care (Pentaris, 2018).

This is also enhanced by Dinham's and Francis's (2015) work, in which they highlight that religious literacy is not acquired simply by getting to know more about more. It would be utopian to expect that hospice professionals, or anyone for that matter, would be able to have in-depth knowledge and understanding of every religion and belief system in the world. Religious literacy is concerned with being comfortable about religion and belief, as well as asking the right questions and working with service users' identities.

Knowledge exchange among hospice staff

In their study about the cultural challenges of hospice staff in Stockholm, Ekblad, Marttila and Emilsson (2000) argued that professionals, both intentionally and unintentionally, engage with each other in group discussions, or on a one-on-one level, to share experiences and knowledge. The researchers argued that this is one of the most effective ways in which professionals advanced their expertise whilst in practise. Like Ekblad, Marttila and Emilsson's argument, this book both presents the case that hospice professionals appear to appreciate deeply the gradual expansion of their knowledge about religion and belief due to exchanges with other staff members, and argues that this is a very effective method of increasing literacy in end of life care.

However, it would be naive of us to accept blindly that this is always the case. Research on burnout and compassion fatigue (e.g., Alkema, Linton and Davies, 2008) suggests that hospice professionals often seek self-care strategies or activities outside of the hospice and work environment. This also means that to avoid the risk of burnout, hospice professionals may be choosing to avoid ongoing engagement with colleagues, especially if group discussions among staff members and knowledge exchange are not mandatory activities or tasks, but a personal choice which materialises outside of the work schedule.

Regardless, and to return to the previous point, the experience of knowledge exchange has been identified by most hospice professionals in Pentaris (2016) as a support system that can only benefit service users. Professionals may often consider seeking extra information from colleagues an essential tool in their work. This is a well-established and frequently necessary principle in hospice care; however, it does come with some complications. Knowledge exchange primarily takes place as an *information transaction*. Mere facts of religious practise are hardly enough evidence to understand a service user's understanding and meaning of life and death. Similarly, information based on the past experiences of other hospice staff are narratives of the professional's life, not a pure representation of a service user's beliefs. This poses questions and ethical dilemmas around what informed-based practise may be and how it should be shaped. It also raises concerns over whether informed-based practise is not necessarily evidence based but is rather purely subjective knowledge, as described by Crisp (2008).

Furthermore, information transactions fail, by their nature, to explore the deep meaning of the data, whereas the same piece of information is the result of the professional's experience in relation to, for example, a dying service user's religion. This fails to consider believing as a unique experience within individual consciousness. The latter was also underlined by Berger (1999), when he changed his position against religion and belief in the public sphere, and suggested that religion and belief have always been present, both in individual consciousness and the public sphere. Belief has no universal example of practise. It is a unique and individualised experience which would be communicated from one professional to another with difficulty, unless the professional's role was to dedicate time and space for rapport building and working through sessions for some period with the service user.

Increased knowledge by professional setting

In line with the previous discussion, it seems a sustained perception that working in a hospice is, in itself, a method of increasing one's knowledge about religion, belief and spirituality. This may seem a logical view when exploring the Christian foundations of hospice care, but it is also a view that is, can, or should be highly contested today. In Chapter 4 I discussed the tendency to mould the space in hospices into a more neutral environment with the intention of making it more inclusive. Although this is taking effect, it seems unlikely that the same environment which is stripped of religious and spiritual references will contribute to the development of professionals' knowledge.

Hospice professionals appear to consider religion, belief and spiritual identities to be related to hospice care and support at the end of life. Furthermore, hospice professionals with more than 15 years of experience in end of life care project the assumption that practising in a hospice environment naturally

---

Box 6.1

'Working within palliative care you are probably more aware of people's spirituality and that it is not just around religion. Spirituality covers much more than that. I think, maybe if you don't work within this sort of area, you might not have this sort of awareness' (Margarita, age 36).

'Hospice work really helps you know much better about religion and spirituality. I guess if you work here, then you are more likely to know better than a nurse in a hospital for instance' (Carol, age 42).

'Working here helps, I guess. I am definitely more aware because of being employed in palliative care' (Judith, age 27).

'In hospices, due to the setting, you know that people will go in deep conversations about religion because this is what you are supposed to do' (Johannes, age 39).

'Working in hospices you become exposed to even more beliefs and even more traditions than you have been exposed previously. So, your knowledge expands' (Cirik, age 46).

---

leads individuals towards development of their knowledge in the areas of religion, belief and spirituality. It seems to me that we are at a turning point. Hospice care, in general derived from Christianity, and professionals who engaged with this field in the past did so either due to religious reasons or with the intention of being led by religion in their work. However, especially since the millennium, hospice care has experienced attempts to neutralise it from religion (discussed earlier) and, therefore, professionals who joined over the last 10 or 15 years do not necessarily share these views.

In summary, hospice professionals seem to suggest that working in end of life care, and hospice care specifically, puts them in a position either to have more opportunities, with regards to spirituality and religion development, or provides the space for a better understanding of why these aspects of life are important (Box 6.1). Indeed, there is a strong link between caring for the dying and/or the bereaved, and the understanding of religion and belief (Golsworthy and Coyle, 2001). Nonetheless, there is no evidence showing that this understanding of religion and belief refers to a general comprehension of belief or faith rather than the personal beliefs of hospice professionals (also see Crisp, 2008).

Understanding of religion and belief

Regardless of the length and breadth of one's knowledge, it needs be coupled with strong understanding and eventual integration of that understanding into professional practise. Research shows (Crisp, 2008) that spirituality is a lived experience which professionals consider as subjective knowledge in helping professions. That said, current professional status that tends to stem from a secular-minded educational background may be contradictory to Crisp's work, though. Despite the contrary evidence, religious literacy, as well as subjective knowledge, are context bound; they can only be appreciated and understood through the context in which they are experienced.

Lack of understanding

Despite the wealth of knowledge and information which hospice professionals acquire, there is evidence that suggests they lack understanding of religion and belief as concepts. Gunaratnam (2001) provides one example. In her work, she critically appraised the exchanges between patients and hospice staff to understand better the context in which they happen and, subsequently, hospice staff's understanding of patients' culture and ethnicity. This example is relevant as Gunaratnam, like many other scholars, has treated culture either as an equal to religion or a subordinate of it, whilst exploring issues of ethnicity in her work. The next example is my research (Pentaris, 2016) in the area of end of life care, which is reflected in this book. Specifically, this study showed a lack of understanding of different faiths, religions and beliefs, inclusive of nonreligion, nonbelief, atheism and agnosticism.

Simultaneously, the difference between different religions is found to be *obscured* or *out of the ordinary*. Of course, this suggests that a sense of logic has been created and adopted by professionals, and anything outside of that logic seems strange and alien. To understand this better, I draw on Northrop's (1947) brilliant collection of essays, which contributed to a much-needed dialogue between social sciences and humanities. Northrop's work emphasised the place of logic in these fields, but also the way these fields generate logic for each other. What Northrop emphasises further is that what is logic, or otherwise normative, is not merely the product of science, but also of everyday life, as well as the arts.

The same study (Pentaris, 2016) presents some further, ground-breaking knowledge in this area. Hospice professionals are not only found to perceive religion, belief and spirituality as concepts which exist in a binary – ordinary and out-of-the-ordinary, but also are found to scrutinise religions and beliefs other than Christianity more critically, recommending that not all are appropriate in a hospice environment due to their *odd nature*. There are many questions arising from this. Most important, do hospice professionals act based on an additional binary (i.e., appropriate and non-appropriate religions)?

In addition, this information leads to further misconceptions and misunderstandings of faith in general. Often, less commonly addressed religions and beliefs are taken as 'weird' or are not acknowledged as religions or faith, but as traditional practises. McGuire (2008) wrote about traditional belief and lived religion extensively. In her book, she examines how the conceptual parts of a belief are carried out through practise and embodiment. However, there is a difference between identifying practises and rituals as the ways faith is expressed (also see Wuthnow, 2012) and interpreting faith

Box 6.2

'Sometimes patients have beliefs that do not make sense. We had a request from a patient from Brighton to come to the hospice here to London to die. He lived all his life in Brighton, and we just went, "Well, why?" And the patient was of the Baha'i faith, and their belief is that after somebody dies, they must be buried at a distance no farther than 50 kilometres from where they died. And, so, they were asking for him to come here, so that he could die here and then be buried in a Baha'i cemetery. In Baha'i religion, there were no kilometres at the time. So, kilometres came out in the 18th century. So, how they managed to measure the distance and bury them in 50 kilometres, I do not know' (Jeremiah, age 58).

'So many faiths I have seen, strange ones ... and ... the beliefs and practises are so not normal as we know them' (Carl, age 51).

'Practices like Mecca are just traditions. Those are not religious practises, like prayer, so we will accommodate as we can but not to an extreme' (Nick, age 41).

'There was this particular situation, the person's ... there was a family and the wife had cancer, and it was felt that the husband's, how to put it, unfaith-fulness to her had somehow angered ... she had become unwell with black magic. And the husband's fear was that if she died, and he was hoping that she would not, her father would be very, very angry and would come to England where they were living and would kill him. No matter how many times we have told him that this is never going to happen and that there is no black magic, he kept believing it, you know' (Carlita, age 46).

as the practise itself. The latter comes with many risks, and I have written about them elsewhere (Pentaris, 2018).

Before we conclude this section, it is worth returning to its initial point: Hospice staff lack an understanding of religion and belief as concepts (Box 6.2). This is neither surprising nor difficult to comprehend. Hage et al. (2006), when exploring counselling and multi-culturalism, put emphasis on professionals' responsibility not only to learn more, but also to use supervision to improve their understanding and appreciation of how religion and belief impact on a person's life. The same argument is presented here; the acquisition of more knowledge is not enough. Hospice staff, and professionals practising across settings in which end of life care is accessible, should widen the way they appreciate the functional roles religion plays in individuals' lives. This will better prepare practitioners to employ a person-centred approach which starts from the individual.

Religion sets boundaries

Similar to Cadge, Ecklund and Short (2009), this study found that hospice professionals experience religion, belief and spirituality both as a barrier to care and also a bridge between individuals and their care. I find the perception of religion, belief and spirituality as a barrier somewhat concerning. The term 'barrier' has a negative connotation which highlights a problematic situation. If one's faith is a barrier to delivering care, does this also mean that the responsibility for this barrier is being placed on the patient or service user? Why should we place responsibility on anyone? Is the ultimate goal of care to show its fullest and best services at all times, or to demonstrate adaptability according to individual needs and preferences? Such questions become pertinent in this situation and they each warrant adequate exploration in future research.

Research puts a lot more emphasis on how religion, spirituality or any faith may inform people's decisions about whether to access and receive hospice care (e.g., Pentaris et al., 2018), a theme discussed in Chapter 5.

The tendency of hospice professionals to consider religion, belief and spirituality a barrier to their practise is also connected with Rothblum's 'Fear of Failure' (1990). Societies have moved towards demanding individuals be high achievers, causing them to experience anxiety of success. This means that anything which prevents success – in this case, complete and elaborate care for every individual, which necessitates standardised care, or otherwise not person-centred – could also be perceived as 'the enemy'. If religion and belief inform decisions which may be incompatible with clinical, medical or allied practise, professionals may experience anxiety and fear of failure. It may be the nature of the helping profession that hospice professionals experience failure when accepting the death of a patient (Bern-Klug, 2010) and it might also indicate resilience toward different approaches in dying.

Skills and abilities to engage with religion and belief

This section focusses on hospice professionals' skills and abilities in engaging with religion and belief. Similar to what Walter (1997) identified as the three approaches of spiritual care in hospice care, this book recognises the role of chaplaincy in hospices when offering spiritual care. In general, the way hospice professionals appear to respond to religion, belief and spiritual needs is by referral to the chaplaincy team. If no one is available in the chaplaincy team, then support is outsourced to the religious network in the community.

Although I recognise the valuable contribution of chaplains in end of life care, I am more interested in exploring how hospice professionals can facilitate faith as a concept which helps people make sense of their experience, rather than how religiously informed demands or preferences are addressed. I am aware that such a statement may not be well received by all disciplines and sciences, but I appreciate that it is open for debate.

Pragmatic approaches

Regardless of whether the professional is a clinical one, hospice professionals, on a 100% tie in Pentaris (2016), are willing to ask what religion people

have, or affiliate with, for a number of reasons. Amongst the most important ones are, initially, asking about religion and belief because legislation
requires it and it is indicated in health policies. This reflects organisational
theories – specifically, bureaucratic and technocratic theories (Hughes and
Wearing, 2017). Hospices may be seen as machines that run as a business
that is achievement focussed and outcomes based. That said, hospice professionals may often find themselves following guidelines that have been
designed for that purpose. Another reason which makes the question 'Do
you have a religion and, if so, what is it?' so paramount to practise is that
the answer becomes an indicator of care, answering pragmatic questions
surrounding the care of the individual (e.g., diet). Last, asking about religion
and belief is a means of avoiding potential harm in the form of spiritual
distress to the service user. The latter was included in the analysis by Boston
and Mount (2006). Palliative professionals in their study aimed towards
minimizing existential and spiritual distress by addressing or attempting to
address religion, belief and spiritual identities.

It is worth noting here the method in which hospice professionals ask about
religion, belief and spirituality. By and large, hospice staff recognises the
subject as highly sensitive and hard-to-reach. Therefore, it is common practise for this subject to be approached primarily once patients or service users
have brought it up themselves. For the purposes of the study which informs
this book (Pentaris, 2016), I spent time reviewing intake or initial interview
forms. The question about religion or belief was left unanswered in over
70% of the cases. This may mean various things; perhaps, patients/service
users decided not to discuss the topic or, and according to the information
presented earlier in this section, hospice professionals were uncomfortable
bringing it up and hence skipped the question. The latter seems more logical,
given the information in this book, and we return to this point in Chapter 8.

Furthermore, my study indicated that religion, belief and spiritual identities are not the priority when patients are admitted. This has a twofold implication. First and foremost, it underlines the prevalence of medical models of
end of life care in general, as well as the bio-medical approaches employed
by hospice professionals and organisational foundations (also described
in my critical analysis [Pentaris, 2013]). Second, itemising the gaining of
knowledge relevant to service users' faiths and belief systems undermines
their dignity as it also indicates lack of respect of someone's preferences in
care (also see Pentaris, 2018; Sue, 2010).

In the extracts in Box 6.3, what is striking is that aspects of belief, faith,
religion, spirituality and so forth all come across as deliberately secondary matters. This is largely questionable, however. Hospice care is developed around the psychosocial and emotional care of an individual, for
whom treatment and medical interventions are no longer an option (also see
Saunders, 2005). If the priority in hospice care is of a medical nature and is
treatment centred or medication centred, what we are left with is, dare I say,
a failed attempt to define hospice care. The WHO's definition of end of life

Box 6.3

'It would always be asked in any transition, any admission, and it is sort of like what their religious beliefs are, you know? That will always be asked. That can have direct affect to their healthcare – for example, with blood transfusions, etc.' (Jeffrey, age 39).

'Jewish people do this and that and you know, obviously I have lots of experience, but I cannot rely on that so much, because it is so different from every individual family – how they express their tradition – so it is just about asking the family and the patient, making clear ... things that have implication for their care' (Carol, age 42).

'Of course, we will ask [the patients], but also you have to wait 'til [the patients] tell you that it is the right time to do so. Otherwise, you might be upsetting someone. I would definitely ask them if they would like to be asked' (Janice, age 47).

'Definitely we will ask, but it is not the first thing to ask, and to be honest it might not be touched at all. I mean, it is not the most important thing when someone is admitted. If it is not brought up in the conversation, then there is no need to explore more at that point' (Michael, age 43).

care has as its core the enhancement of quality of life, whilst specifying that prolonging life is not the aim. The definition also adds that spiritual aspects of care should be integrated. This is one of the examples that illustrate the contradiction and controversies with this study – a metamorphosis of *hospice care* to *hospice cure*.

Of course, this is not to generalise widely across all hospice professionals, but to emphasise a practise and mindset which appears to prevail. Having said that, there appears to be a difference between generations in relation to asking about religion, belief and spiritual identities. Younger professionals who participated in this study expressed the view that, to avoid assumptions about an individual's preference, perception and lifestyle, one should always ask them. However, older professionals do not express such ideas or exemplify them.

This may be an indicator of the education received by different generations, at various times, and in relation to the shifting role of religion in the public space (also see Chapters 2 and 5). Nonetheless, older individuals that do not refer to these notions have had longstanding experience with hospice care. On the contrary, younger professionals have practised in hospice care for a very short period. Perhaps this gap in experience between generations is also influential.

Figure 6.2 depicts the reasons why professionals would seek knowledge of the service users' religious or nonreligious belief and practise, by profession. Two categories emerge from this: *pragmatic* and *understanding*. Hospice professionals ask individuals what their religion, belief and spiritual identities are, mainly, as shown in Figure 6.2, due to pragmatic reasons.

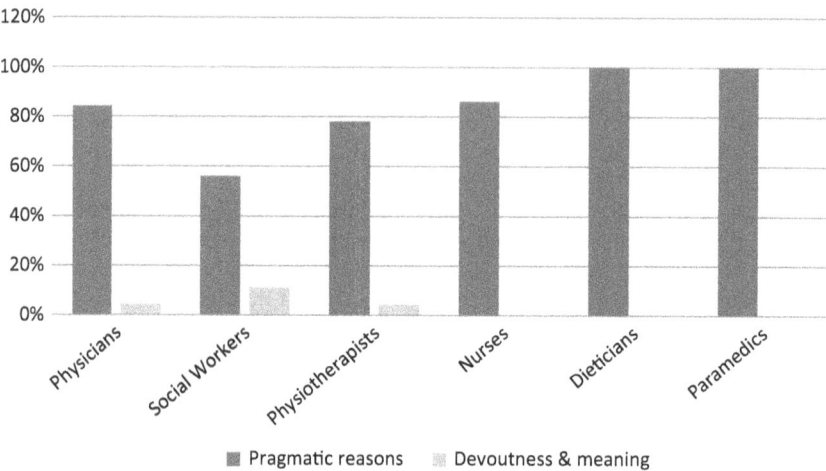

Figure 6.2 Reasons for asking about religion and belief by profession

Examples of these are food preferences, gender match (e.g., female professional with female patient), funeral preparations, visitation style and arrangements (e.g., how many people and for how long). On the contrary, only a small number of professionals, mostly social workers, with smaller numbers of physicians and physiotherapists, ask religious- or belief-related questions to understand how the patient/service user is experiencing their dying, imminent death, and/or grief and bereavement.

Devoutness, or level of belief or nonbelief is, in general, not, overall, an aspect of someone's life that hospice professionals will register, or seek knowledge about. This results in lack of insight into the individual's meaning-making process (also see Park, 2013). In addition, this frustrates the 'spiritual care' aims in end of life and hospice care. Furthermore, Figure 6.2 raises the issue that hospice practise is primarily interested in collecting information about religious practise and religious-centred traditions of the patients/service users. Although important, such practise perhaps defies the principles of holistic care and approaches (Sepúlveda et al., 2002), as well as the NHS Constitution (launched in March 2013), that presents suggestions about dignity and respect for the individual, compassionate care and informed choice of service users.

Religious/Spiritual Care Toolkit

It seems an absolute necessity for hospices either to develop or to adopt an existing *spiritual care tool*. Gordon and Mitchell (2004) identified the lack of definition of spiritual care or validation of a spiritual assessment tool, and proposed a competence-based approach to delivering spiritual care. In other words, the authors recommended that spiritual care may be delivered by any professional in the field, based on their competence to do so.

What this section uncovers is an opposing ideology to Gordon and Mitchell's (2004) work. The use of a tool, applicable in all cases, which presents a fixed questionnaire also suggests that all staff have the competence to collect the information about religion or belief, but without special training, awareness or expertise.

Of course, a spiritual care tool is neither uncommon nor unnecessary. However, the validity of the tool, as well as the way it is used in practise, play a critical role in the success of spiritual care. Often, hospice professionals employ tools which have been validated to be effective in practise, but do not always have adequate training to use them effectively. An example is the Grupo de Espiritualidad de la SECPAL questionnaire (Spanish Society of Palliative Care [SECPAL] Task Force on Spiritual Care) (Benito et al., 2014). This tool uses initial questions to build rapport with a service user, leading to questions aimed at developing a concrete understanding of the service user's religion, belief or spirituality and what it means to them. Another example is the FICA Tool (Faith & Belief, Importance, Community, and Address in Care) for Spiritual Assessment (Borneman, Ferrell and Puchalski, 2010). This tool is designed to explore faith or belief, the importance of spirituality, the individual's spiritual community and interventions to address spiritual needs. Once again, this example shows that spiritual care tools are necessary and effective (Johnson, 2001).

This section, however, does not focus on tools designed for spiritual assessment (a discussion about those is available in Pentaris [2018]). It highlights the common practise of using an, often in-house, spiritual care tool that may have not been tested and validated to ensure effective spiritual care, given that spiritual care begins with spiritual assessment (Box 6.4) (also see Puchalski and Romer, 2000). Also, this section reveals that spiritual care tools that lack validation or have not been piloted are often simple questionnaires, which may be filled in by the service user or not – in other words, tools which lack the emotionality described by Benito et al. (2014) and, therefore, the ability to offer the chance for building rapport between hospice staff and service users.

Box 6.4

'We have a spiritual care tool, but I think it is just very recently that it started to be used' (Mirna, age 48).

'All the tools in spiritual care help us talk about religion with patients, or not exactly talk about it, but at least we note it down' (John, age 53).

'There are definitely forms that religion is included in them. I mean, we ask people, but of course only if they are able to answer' (Dorothy, age 37).

'Simple thing, when we do the initial assessment with all patients, we always ask about physiological stuff like the food they prefer, but then it is the meaning that their choice has to them. The cultural, religious aspects of food. So, that is part of that assessment' (Anna, age 59).

Professional knowledge

Benner (1984) emphasised the need for further development of competencies in nursing, echoing a consensus across health and social care disciplines. Attard, Baldacchino and Camilleri (2014) drew on Benner's work and suggested that the same approach can be applied to spiritual care. Using a competency-based approach with healthcare professionals, it is highly likely that the ability to provide spiritual care will increase. There are, however, many challenges that come with this. Who has identified the 'right' competencies necessary to provide spiritual care? When were they identified and do they fit into the ever-changing socio-political context in which hospice care is provided? For whom are these competencies identified? Do they refer to one discipline over another?

Similarly to Gordon and Mitchell's (2004) work, the competency-based approach is focused on ability, but more emphasis should be given to perception. Without an accurate perception of circumstances, it is unlikely that abilities would be put to good use. In other words, a competency-based model seems, to me, a more practical choice and it leaves professionals exposed due to a possible lack of self-awareness in this area.

Aside from the argument about competency versus perception, it is evident in practise that hospice professionals appreciate engagement with the religion, belief and spiritual identities of service users, based on the individual professional's skills and knowledge (Pentaris, 2016). Whether and how one responds to needs related to religion or belief is therefore dependent on individual practise.

A point worth mentioning arises from Pentaris (2016): Individual hospice professionals suggest that their skills and abilities are dependent on their unique knowledge. This supports the argument that it is not possible to generalise findings of hospice professionals being religiously illiterate or uncomfortable engaging with religion, belief, and spiritual identities. On the other hand, and back to the point about who identifies which competencies are the right ones, professionals appear to use their own personal judgement during initial assessments to understand how service users position themselves in relation to religion and belief. This argument ties in well with Day's (2011) work in relation to what people mean by belonging. Often, information is retrieved regarding religious or nonreligious affiliation, but what that actually entails in the service user's life remains undiscussed. When professionals use their own judgement to decide whether service users are devout or have needs relating to that aspect of their lives, they also run the risk of misjudging the circumstances. In Williams et al. (2011), it becomes apparent that many patients do not have the opportunity to discuss religion or belief with healthcare professionals, despite the abundant research that suggests how the former impacts on the quality of care service users receive. What comes across from the study by Williams et al. (2011) is that professionals do not always suggest that having a discussion about religion is necessary with

---

Box 6.5

'Whether patients are devout – we would couple that again within their spirituality. So, their devoutness would come into it. Quite often, when people give you their religion you usually get some sort of flavour as to how devout they are' (Raul, age 26).

'When you are doing the assessment, you quite understand whether patients are devout to their religion or not. They give it away at the time of asking them their religious affiliation' (Jeffrey, age 39).

---

all patients. This is compatible with findings from Pentaris (2016), in which it is evident that hospice professionals often 'make the call' on whether a service user wants to talk about religion or belief (Box 6.5).

To return to the initial point about relying on self-identified knowledge and skills, this is increasingly worrying for several reasons. First and foremost, the education received by hospice professionals (or healthcare professionals in general) across disciplines is dubious in terms of universal content when it comes to religion and belief. This also raises issues with assessment and evaluation of the services, which seem hard to achieve if services are bound by an individual perception or stance. Also, it brings ethical issues to the surface, such as lack of equity in hospice care. According to Coward and Stajduhar (2012), hospice care has always been concerned with ethical issues in relation to how well-prepared practitioners are to care for the dying and the bereaved. In addition, a professional's perception of whether religion or belief are important aspects of life might signify their engagement with service users. In other words, the reliance on personal perception may distort the ideal of person-centred hospice care.

Personal beliefs in the professional

An important point to consider is the following: Hospice professionals often understand personal beliefs and religion to be key factors towards better understanding of the target group in hospice care. The perception that personal beliefs, which are integrated into professional practise, only enhance the chances for more developed skills and abilities in this area, is depicted in the extracts in Box 6.6.

It is also suggested here that hospice professionals should have religious belief to engage with the religion, belief, and spiritual identities of service users. Over 20 years ago, Millison and Dudley (1990) reported that hospice professionals who are more spiritual and/or religious seem to experience higher job satisfaction. Equally, the relationship between personal spirituality and practising in a hospice was highlighted by Sinclair's (2011) work. Sinclair proposed that working in a hospice enables professionals to seek spiritual growth and

> **Box 6.6**
>
> 'I think having a belief system, for me personally, does help with looking after this group of patients, and to be able to face it on a day-to-day basis and to give the support that is needed to the relatives in particular' (Mirna, age 48).
>
> 'One of our junior doctors was a devout Muslim, and I do not know how ... we had a Turkish patient, who had just died, and I do not know why, the patient's wife ran up to him and said, 'My husband has just died. Can you please come in and say a prayer at his bedside?' (Jeremiah, age 58).
>
> 'Being neutral about this myself actually helps me being open-minded to all different cultures and religions that I come across with. I don't believe in anything, so it is easier to talk about anything' (Judith, age 27).

satisfaction for themselves, whilst alluding to the fact that spiritual growth then empowers professionals to continue caring for the dying and bereaved. This is also not far from the conception of hospice care (see Chapter 1), which is intertwined with professionals' religious and/or spiritual identity.

In addition to this point, hospice professionals present the belief that being a Christian, specifically, is vital for understanding and working within a religiously diverse environment (Box 6.7). This matches Zuckerman's (2008) recommendation that 'being Christian' appears to mean "being kind to others and taking care of the poor and sick"'. Yet, it seems to me that such ideas may present barriers to the enhancement of spiritual/religious care among hospice professionals who may not be Christian, or may be of no faith. A similar example is seen in Callahan (2015). The author suggested that Christian social workers have an additional source of support when practising in hospices: Christianity. However, Callahan did not exclude the potential of social workers with a different faith or none. It is very interesting to see how religious belief drives hospice professionals towards their professionalism. However, this might not match the expectations or desires of a service user who is either non-Christian or nonreligious.

> **Box 6.7**
>
> 'I am totally able to engage with religious identities, because I am a Christian by belief. I believe there is a God and a son of God, and I knew before I came to this hospice that it was a multi-faith, no faith – it was everything. And part of my role is to meet people where they are at. So, I have no problem with any of that at all. I am here to meet people where they are at and help them if I can' (Carol, age 42).
>
> 'I am a good Christian, so I know how to respond to other beliefs too' (John, age 53).

Chaplains

An additional practise which hospice professionals appear to identify as a skill of religious literacy is the way in which they collaborate with chaplains, when available. Many scholars before now (e.g., Kelley and Morrison, 2015; Fitchett et al., 2011; Greer et al., 2013) have examined both the relationship between chaplains and other palliative professionals, and the role of the chaplains in delivering spiritual care. Kelley and Morrison (2015) particularly focussed on comparing physicians' and chaplains' views about the role of the chaplain in paediatric palliative care. The consensus from this study was that chaplains are the solely responsible practitioners for meeting religion-, belief- and spirituality-related service user needs. This finding has, of course, been contested, not only in western countries (e.g., McSherry, 2001), but also in Asia (Mok, Wong and Wong, 2010).

This section however, does not focus on the role of chaplains in the delivery of hospice and palliative care. It reports on information which further suggests that referring service users to the chaplaincy team is a very common practise which not only masks religious illiteracy, but also presents as controversial. To explain the latter further, hospice professionals, as has been discussed in Chapters 5 and 6, suggest that they acquire advanced, or at least adequate, knowledge and skills to support service users' needs relating to religion or belief. Referring service users to the chaplaincy team, however, when such needs arise, could mean either that professionals lack the religious literacy to explore such aspects of the person's care further, or consider the ability to make such referrals part and parcel with religious literacy.

Findings from Pentaris (2016) are also controversial and contradictory. Despite the highly regarded self-perception of skills and abilities for engagement with individuals' religion and belief, hospice professionals select a practical solution on what I like to call a *spiritual care emergency kit* (Table 6.1).

Whether I have challenged the following in earlier chapters, it is still appropriate to say that spiritual care is integral to psychosocial support – a task primarily delivered by social workers and sometimes nurses or other healthcare professionals, but not by chaplains (Reese and Brown, 1997; also see Haugk, 1976). McSherry (2001), on the other hand, revisits the traditional role of nurses, which he claims is to be spiritual carers. His suggestion is based on the historical development of nursing from within religious institutions and medieval Christianity. On the contrary, Nolan (2012) challenges McSherry's (2001, p. 118) views, amongst others, when he claims that the role of spiritual carer 'is more suited to that of a suitably qualified spiritual advisor or guide'. Even though Nolan's critique lacks clarity and evidence to be considered in the way the spiritual care emergency kit works, it is, however, the dominant practise observed.

Table 6.1 Spiritual care emergency kit

Participants' responses

- If someone needs spiritual support or religious support, we can always be available to call the chaplain of the hospice (Michael, age 43).
- I will always contact the chaplaincy team if a patient seems more religious, if they seem to require more support spiritually (John, age 53).
- Patients can always be referred to the chaplain if they have any spiritual needs, like their religion (Shahid, age 33).
- Even if the person is not well, and the relatives have informed us about the patient's religion, we will bring in a religious leader from their own group (Dorothy, age 37).
- I tell patients that if they want to talk about [religion], I can find someone to come and talk to them. Possibly from the chaplaincy team (Carlita, age 46).
- There is always a list with the contact numbers of the chaplains in the office, so if needed we can look it up there (Mark, age 61).
- Yes, we are very comfortable with this [in this hospice]. We share this information with colleagues during MDT meetings. Like, if someone has spiritual needs, we will say that we need to call, I do not know, the Church of England minister, or X chaplain (Nick, age 41).
- Efforts are made to facilitate [service users'] own pastor or specific religious leader to come in. Alternatively, there are many people in the community who are able to be called upon and come in and run last rites and do whatever specific religions do (Mirna, age 48).
- In this hospice, they have a chaplaincy here, and they have a Roman Catholic and they have a Church of England on staff. They also have other people … a list of people who are called in, and it is led by one of the nuns (Carl, age 51).

References

Alkema, K., Linton, J.M. and Davies, R., 2008. A study of the relationship between self-care, compassion satisfaction, compassion fatigue, and burnout among hospice professionals. *Journal of Social Work in End-of-Life & Palliative Care*, 4(2), pp. 101–119.

Attard, J., Baldacchino, D.R. and Camilleri, L., 2014. Nurses' and midwives' acquisition of competency in spiritual care: A focus on education. *Nurse Education Today*, 34(12), pp. 1460–1466.

Ayer, A.J. and Marić, S., 1956. *The problem of knowledge* (pp. 173–175). Harmondsworth: Penguin Books.

Benito, E., Oliver, A., Galiana, L., Barreto, P., Pascual, A., Gomis, C. and Barbero, J., 2014. Development and validation of a new tool for the assessment and spiritual care of palliative care patients. *Journal of Pain and Symptom Management*, 47(6), pp. 1008–1018.

Benner, P., 1984. *From novice to expert*. Menlo Park, CA: Addison-Wesley.

Berger, P.L., 1999. The desecularization of the world: A global overview. In Berger, P.L. (ed.), *The desecularization of the world: Resurgent religion and world politics*. Washington, DC: William B. Eerdmans, pp. 1–18.

Bern-Klug, M. (ed.), 2010. *Transforming palliative care in nursing homes: The social work role*. New York, NY: Columbia University Press.

Borneman, T., Ferrell, B. and Puchalski, C.M., 2010. Evaluation of the FICA tool for spiritual assessment. *Journal of Pain and Symptom Management*, 40(2), pp. 163–173.

Boston, P.H. and Mount, B.M., 2006. The caregiver's perspective on existential and spiritual distress in palliative care. *Journal of Pain and Symptom Management*, 32(1), pp. 13–26.

Cadge, W., Ecklund, E.H. and Short, N., 2009. Religion and spirituality: A barrier and a bridge in the everyday professional work of pediatric physicians. *Social Problems*, 56(4), pp. 702–721.

Callahan, A.M., 2015. Key concepts in spiritual care for hospice social workers: How an interdisciplinary perspective can inform spiritual competence. *Social Work and Christianity*, 42(1), pp. 43–62.

Campbell, C.D., 1971. *Toward a sociology of irreligion*. London: Macmillan.

Coward, H. and Stajduhar, K.I. (eds.), 2012. *Religious understandings of a good death in hospice palliative care*. New York, NY: State University New York Press.

Crisp, B.R., 2008. Social work and spirituality in a secular society. *Journal of Social Work*, 8(4), pp. 363–375.

Daaleman, T.P. and VandeCreek, L., 2000. Placing religion and spirituality in end-of-life care. *Journal of the American Medical Association*, 284(19), pp. 2514–2517.

Davie, G., 2015. *Religion in Britain: A persistent paradox*. Oxford, UK: Wiley-Blackwell.

Day, A., 2011. *Believing in belonging: Belief and social identity in the modern world*. Oxford, UK: Oxford University Press.

Dinham, A. and Francis, M. (eds.), 2015. *Religious literacy in policy and practice*. Bristol, UK: Policy Press.

Ekblad, S., Marttila, A. and Emilsson, M., 2000. Cultural challenges in end-of-life care: Reflections from focus groups' interviews with hospice staff in Stockholm. *Journal of Advanced Nursing*, 31(3), pp. 623–630.

Feagin, J., 2013. *Systemic racism: A theory of oppression*. London, UK: Routledge.

Fitchett, G., Lyndes, K.A., Cadge, W., Berlinger, N., Flanagan, E. and Misasi, J., 2011. The role of professional chaplains on pediatric palliative care teams: Perspectives from physicians and chaplains. *Journal of Palliative Medicine*, 14(6), pp. 704–707.

Golsworthy, R. and Coyle, A., 2001. Practitioners' accounts of religious and spiritual dimensions in bereavement therapy. *Counselling Psychology Quarterly*, 14(3), pp. 183–202.

Gordon, T. and Mitchell, D., 2004. A competency model for the assessment and delivery of spiritual care. *Palliative Medicine*, 18(7), pp. 646–651.

Greer, J.A., Jackson, V.A., Meier, D.E. and Temel, J.S., 2013. Early integration of palliative care services with standard oncology care for patients with advanced cancer. *CA: A Cancer Journal for Clinicians*, 63(5), pp. 349–363.

Gunaratnam, Y., 2001. Eating into multiculturalism: Hospice staff and service users talk food, 'race', ethnicity, culture and identity. *Critical Social Policy*, 21(3), pp. 287–310.

Hage, S.M., Hopson, A., Siegel, M., Payton, G. and DeFanti, E., 2006. Multicultural training in spirituality: An interdisciplinary review. *Counseling and Values*, 50(3), pp. 217–234.

Haugk, K.C., 1976. Unique contributions of churches and clergy to community mental health. *Community Mental Health Journal*, 12(1), pp. 20–28.

Hermann, C., 2000. A guide to the spiritual needs of elderly cancer patients. *Geriatric Nursing*, 21(6), pp. 324–325.

Hook, J.N., Davis, D.E., Owen, J., Worthington Jr., E.L. and Utsey, S.O., 2013. Cultural humility: Measuring openness to culturally diverse clients. *Journal of Counseling Psychology*, 60(3), pp. 353–366.

Hughes, M. and Wearing, M., 2017. *Organisations and management in social work*. Thousand Oaks, CA: Sage.

Johnson, C.P., 2001. Assessment tools: Are they an effective approach to implementing spiritual health care within the NHS? *Accident and Emergency Nursing*, 9(3), pp. 177–186.

Kelley, A.S. and Morrison, R.S., 2015. Palliative care for the seriously ill. *New England Journal of Medicine*, 373(8), pp. 747–755.

Knowles, E.D. and Peng, K., 2005. White selves: Conceptualizing and measuring a dominant-group identity. *Journal of Personality and Social Psychology*, 89(2), pp. 223–241.

Kronenfeld, J.J. (ed.), 2010. *The impact of demographics on health and health care: Race, ethnicity and other social factors*. London, UK: Emerald.

Li, X., 2004. A case study of interreligious relations in contemporary China: Buddhist–Christian interaction in four southeast cities. *Ching Feng*, 5(1), pp. 93–118.

London, L., 2008. The Church of England and the Holocaust: Christianity, memory and Nazism. *The Catholic Historical Review*, 94(1), pp. 171–173.

McGuire, M.B., 2008. *Lived religion: Faith and practice in everyday life*. Oxford: Oxford University Press.

McSherry, W., 2001. Spiritual crisis? Call a nurse. In Orchard, H. (ed.), *Spirituality in Health Care Contexts*, London, UK: Jessica Kingsley.

Millison, M.B. and Dudley, J.R., 1990. The importance of spirituality in hospice work: A study of hospice professionals. *The Hospice Journal*, 6(3), pp. 63–78.

Mok, E., Wong, F. and Wong, D., 2010. The meaning of spirituality and spiritual care among the Hong Kong Chinese terminally ill. *Journal of Advanced Nursing*, 66(2), pp. 360–370.

Nolan, S., 2012. *Spiritual care at the end of life: The chaplain as a 'Helpful Presence'*. London, UK: Jessica Kingsley.

Northrop, F.S.C., 1947. *The logic of the sciences and the humanities*. London, UK: Macmillan.

O'Connor, P., 1988. The role of spiritual care in hospice: Are we meeting patients' needs? *American Journal of Hospice Care*, 5(4), pp. 31–37.

Park, C.L., 2013. Religion and meaning. In Paloutzian, R.F. and Park, C.L. (eds.), *Handbook of the psychology of religion and spirituality*. New York, NY: Guilford Press, pp. 357–379.

Pentaris, P., 2018. The marginalization of religion in end of life care: Signs of microaggression? *International Journal of Human Rights in Healthcare*, 11(2), pp. 116–128.

Pentaris, P., 2016. *Religious literacy in end of life care: Challenges and controversies*. Unpublished Doctoral Thesis (Goldsmiths, University of London).

Puchalski, C. and Romer, A.L., 2000. Taking a spiritual history allows clinicians to understand patients more fully. *Journal of Palliative Medicine*, 3(1), pp. 129–137.

Reese, D.J. and Brown, D.R., 1997. Psychosocial and spiritual care in hospice: Differences between nursing, social work, and clergy. *The Hospice Journal*, 12(1), pp. 29–41.

Rothblum, E.D., 1990. Fear of failure. In Leitenberg, H. (ed.), *Handbook of social and evaluation anxiety*. New York, NY: Springer Science & Business Media, pp. 497–537.

Saunders, D.C., 2005. *Cicely Saunders – Founder of the Hospice Movement: Selected letters 1959-1999*. Oxford, UK: Oxford University Press.

Sepúlveda, C., Marlin, A., Yoshida, T. and Ullrich, A., 2002. Palliative care: The World Health Organization's global perspective. *Journal of Pain and Symptom Management*, 24(2), pp. 91–96.

Sinclair, S., 2011. Impact of death and dying on the personal lives and practices of palliative and hospice care professionals. *Canadian Medical Association Journal*, 183(2), pp. 180–187.

Smith-Stoner, M., 2007. End-of-life preferences for atheists. *Journal of Palliative Medicine*, 10(4), pp. 923–928.

Sue, D.W., 2010. *Microaggressions in everyday life: Race, gender, and sexual orientation*. London, UK: Wiley.

Walter, T., 1997. The ideology and organization of spiritual care: Three approaches. *Palliative Medicine*, 11(1), pp. 21–30.

Williams, J.A., Meltzer, D., Arora, V., Chung, G. and Curlin, F.A., 2011. Attention to inpatients' religious and spiritual concerns: Predictors and association with patient satisfaction. *Journal of General Internal Medicine*, 26(11), pp. 1265–1271.

Wuthnow, R., 2012. *The God problem: Expressing faith and being reasonable*. Oakland, CA: University of California Press.

Zuckerman, P., 2008. *Society without God: What the least religious nations can tell us about contentment*. New York, NY: NYU Press.

7 Integrating religion and belief in hospice care

Introduction

In the previous chapters of the second part of the book, we specifically examined three areas. First, how religion, belief and spirituality – inclusive of nonreligion, nonbelief and nonspirituality – are represented, or not, in the space of hospices. Next, we delved into an exploration of how hospice professionals perceive and appreciate religion, belief and spirituality. We started from perceptions about religion in the public domain and moved on to discuss perceptions about religion in relation to hospice patients' experiences. Following on from this, we looked at both knowledge and understanding, and skills and abilities of hospice professionals when working with individuals for whom faith, or the lack of, is important. To bring this full circle, it is only natural that we now discuss the ways in which religion, belief and spirituality are integrated aspects of hospice practise. This discussion is the culmination of the second part of the book.

As discussed in Chapter 1, religion, belief and spirituality are essential aspects of care when working with people who are experiencing a terminal illness or bereavement. This is not a ground-breaking statement, but an important one which bears reiterating. Puchalski (2007–2008) also emphasised this, drawing on spiritual care models in the US. Research widely supports that service users in hospice and palliative care, and end of life care more generally, want their spiritual needs (whatever their definition) appreciated and embedded in their care, yet not many people report this to be the case when they have received care (see Puchalski, 2007–2008). The latter remains debatable in practise and research. There is abundant evidence of the initiatives aiming at addressing spiritual care in hospice and palliative care, yet little inquiry about the sustaining ambiguity of the practises, as we shall see later.

The discussion about how religion and belief are integrated in professional practise is a topic explored in many fields, predominantly in clinical practise and psychology. Tan (1996) examined how religion is integrated in psychotherapy and clinical practise more generally, for example. That study highlighted the compatibility of spiritual care with the principles and values of clinical practise – a theme not uncommon to other disciplines, such as social work and nursing. Equally, Young and Young (2014), as well as Wolf and Stevens (2001), explored the integration of religion and spirituality in counselling. The former emphasised the need to provide further methods for spiritual care to enhance the holistic aspect of care. The latter focusses more on both the barriers posed when integrating religion and belief in practise (e.g., limited options in methods of care) and the positives it has, like providing more space for compassionate care.

Many studies have explored professionals' views about the integration of religion and spirituality in practise. An example is Furman et al. (2004), who researched the attitudes of social workers on the subject. Some findings worth noting from that study include the perception that spirituality (and not religion) is a fundamental aspect of the human experience. Also, most social workers in that study reported they had not received any form of training on the subject during their programme of education. Last, and most pertinent to this chapter, social work professionals suggested that considering the aspects of religion, belief and spirituality when working with individuals who experience a terminal illness is paramount.

These are only but a few examples which provide additional emphasis on the ongoing dialogue about whether religion, belief and spirituality should be taken into account in practise. However, not many studies have looked at the ways in which this happens in practise. Aside from the numerous explorations of spiritual care models and their impact, we still do not know how they materialise. Puchalski (2007–2008) offers a helpful typology of spiritual care: *intrinsic* and *extrinsic*. The intrinsic aspect of spiritual care refers to a more compassionate presence of the professional whereas the extrinsic component refers to the more practical ways of addressing spiritual needs, such as dietary requirements. This typology proves very helpful in our discussion in concluding chapter of this book.

Death and health policies

Whether national, local or organisational, policy seems to be taking a toll in the way in which hospice professionals appreciate that religion, belief and spirituality are integrated into their practise. Chapter 3 emphasised this and examined how social policy impacts on practise, and showed that definitional challenges in policy language play out in professional practise as well. My previous work in hospices (Pentaris, 2016) supports this as well. All hospice professionals who partook in Pentaris (2016) recommended that religion and spirituality are both integrated well in professional practise as they are both suggested aspects of care in social policy. In other words, hospice professionals appear to consider integration in social policy equivalent to integration in professional practise (Box 7.1).

Of course, this raises a serious dilemma. Social policy is a frame of communicating the emotionality of legislation (also see Alcock, 2014) – the full length of legal jargon government documents which guide general practise

---

Box 7.1

'Well, [spirituality] has been integrated because it is part of the policies, you know, diversity policies and all that. And also, NHS guidance documents always talk about universal care' (Alex, age 44).

'[Spirituality] is within everything and also policies on diversity. It is prevailing everything and we [professionals] did not see that coming. Religion is part of it as well, so it is very present, and integrated in healthcare' (Cirik, age 46).

'Well, you know, it is in our policy to ask patients [about belief] when they come in. And, you know, it is sort of part of the diversity thing' (Carl, age 51).

---

and social structures. Therefore, social policy providing a framework for practise perhaps highlights the importance of the different aspects of practise and stretches what is *correct* in it. That said, integration on a social policy level does not equate to integration on a professional practise level. The latter would carry out the guidance provided by the social policy by means of models of practise and other methods. With this division in mind, the perception that integration of belief in policy necessitates its integration in practise questions the ability of individual professionals to comprehend social policy documents, or otherwise the organisation's (i.e., hospice) abilities to transcend policies to the employees.

Catto and Perfect (2015) examined the separation of policy and practise as well. In their account, they state that 'following the enactment of the Equality Act 2010, religion or belief is protected specifically in employment and the provision of goods and services in England and Wales' (Catto and Perfect, 2015, p. 135). Yet, the Act only makes the recommendation and communicates legal responsibilities. Whether this is carried out in practise is a separate subject. Professional practise in hospices is also informed by social policy, like Equality Act 2010, to name one. Yet, social policy alone is not sufficient evidence of the integration of religion, belief and spirituality in professional practise. In addition, a policy's inability to measure the methods by which its content is carried out in practise places more space between delivery of and the need to deliver care related to people's religion, belief and spiritual needs.

Assessments

An alternative way which hospice professionals describe as a method of integrating religion, belief and spirituality in practise is assessment work, and – more specifically – the initial assessment when someone is admitted to a hospice. Hospice professionals, regardless of their disciplinary background, support that enquiring about a person's religion or belief during the initial assessment is solid proof of the former being well embedded in professional practise (Pentaris, 2016). To understand this better, I engaged with research participants in a more in-depth discussion about this topic.

Box 7.2

'Proof of that is that we do the initial assessment with all patients, and the initial assessment includes a question about religion' (Michael, age 43).

'The initial assessment, which is done by nurses and doctors, also asks questions about spiritual beliefs and religion. So, religion has been integrated, I guess' (Shahid, age 33).

'When a person is admitted, that person is asked about his or her religion or faith or spirituality; and, if the patient is too unwell to speak, we often ask the relatives' (Johannes, age 39).

'We always ask people when they are admitted' (John, age 53).

'What, generally, healthcare does is that they usually ask it as a certain question: What is this person's race? What is this person's religion? And I think this is what we do. It is at a very superficial level, without any real understanding about what that means and without really paying any great care attention' (Nick, age 41).

'In the beginning, we will ask if they have a religion and, if yes, we can contact the right person from that religion' (Mirna, age 48).

'So, we have got a form which will say, 'What is your ethnicity, religion and language?' So, from that we will know what to do at the end' (Alex, age 44).

'We ask patients in the beginning. That is a general practise that the doctor or nurse who are doing it will always remember to ask. If they do not, then at some point someone else will do so' (Gita, age 59).

Of primary concern in this discussion was the need to find out more about how this topic is discussed and under what structure, if any (Box 7.2).

Unlike the suggestion by Daaleman et al. (2008) that professionals in end of life care appear to consider spiritual care delivery as an act of *being present* (equal to the intrinsic aspect of spiritual care [Puchalski, 2007–2008]), professionals in Pentaris (2016) seemed to consider spiritual care delivery a more measured process – one in which they ask people who arrive for hospice care what their religious affiliation is, if any, and whether they want to be connected with the respective religious leader (Box 7.3).

To do this topic better justice, I think a few pointers are in need. First, end of life care is a much wider context than simply hospice care. The former may involve care in the community and in the person's home. Hospice care, on the other hand, even though it could present itself as an outsourced service or delivered in the community as well, mostly refers to the institutionalised care of the dying and support for the bereaved. With that in mind, *being present* may be feasible and far more realistic in community hospice care rather than care in hospice organisations.

An additional point to make here is the separate context in which the previously mentioned data refer to. The work by Daaleman et al. (2008) refers to the US, whereas Pentaris (2016) was informed by perceptions of professionals in the UK. It is imperative to be reminded of the vast differences in

Box 7.3

'When a patient is admitted, a questionnaire is used for assessment. Part of the questions is sort of asking them their name or address, and also their religion. So, it is put down as to what religion they are, and that is how it is looked at' (Nick, age 41).

'There is a question that asks the patients what their language, ethnicity and religion are. We will always tick that box so that we know that the patient has a religion' (Dorothy, age 37).

'In the patient's file, there is always a ticked box if they have told us in the past that they are religious' (Jeremiah, age 58).

'We ask everyone when they are admitted, and we tick a box' (Margarita, age 36).

'Conversation about religion and spirituality takes place at the first contact with the patient, if appropriate. But then, the tick box form is really what will tell [professionals] what the patient wants' (Carlita, age 46).

'There is a box about religion, and if that is ticked, we know that the person has religious needs' (Peter, age 31).

'If someone has ticked the box of religion in the assessment, then we will know to ask patients what they want for their dying' (Carol, age 42).

education, training, conceptions and philosophy of care for any comparison to be successful.

There is a main similarity between this section and the discussion about death and health policies. Considering the integration of religion, belief and spirituality in professional practise as a form of assessment, which seeks to gather information rather than develop or gain an understanding of human experience, highlights the technocratic and bureaucratic culture we often encounter in hospice and palliative care in the UK (Zimmermann, 2012; James and Field, 1992; Reese, Melton and Ciaravino, 2004) and elsewhere (Phillips and Agar, 2016; James and Field, 1992), and which often clashes with professional practise (Pentaris, 2014). This happens either by adding administrative work to the already overwhelming roles of hospice professionals, or by confusing and misleading professionals from their primary role: to provide quality care and promote the wellbeing of the service user. In the debates of secular ideas, it is underlined that religion is privatised and far from public discussion (also see Davie, 2013). Therefore, technocratic approaches in hospice care also seem timely and appropriate, but not necessarily effective.

An example that illustrates the argument of technocracy is the use of itemised forms which are used to record people's aspects of their identity, such as ethnicity or language. The information is later used to inform a patient's care plan. Such practise has both a positive and a challenging outcome. First, also stressed in *Defining Quality in Hospice Care* by Hospice UK (2014), such tools help tease out information necessary to enhance and promote quality of care on the whole. To the contrary, though, and also mentioned in the same report, forms collecting factual information which lack emotion (i.e., what is meant by it) offer outcome measures for use in hospice and palliative care – an evaluation process for successful hospice and palliative care delivery.

Hospice UK (2014) highlighted the various domains of quality of care in hospices and palliative care teams. The domains include spiritual/religious care, as well as information needs for decision-making. To understand better the contrast of itemising characteristics and considering it a form of integration of religion, belief and spirituality in hospice care, one should consider the following example. If a person's religion is noted as Muslim, this satisfied the domain of information needs for decision-making – for example, what the preferences and wishes of the patient are, dietary requirements, and other needs. However, how does this information, which lacks depth and substance regarding the person's experience of religion, inform the domain of spiritual/religious care, unless we accept the latter simply to be met by making a referral to the right religious leader or offer the most appropriate diet?

Hospice professionals in my study (Pentaris, 2016) appear to consider the recording of information about religion or belief a very important task, and it is. Yet, by and large, professionals rarely spend time to unpick the meaning and impact of the information they collect during an initial assessment. This disadvantages the hospice team's understanding of service users' needs, but also leaves the latter in a precarious situation regarding the quality of the care they will receive. Having ticked a box, or filled in a form saying that someone is religious, does not explicitly indicate what that means. Is the service user overly devout and requests daily prayers, or is he or she traditionally religious and shows no relation to the beliefs, values and/or principles of the religion registered in the form? In other words, what does a person's religion, belief or spiritual identity mean to them?

This is reflected in the *vicarious religion* thesis (Davie, 2007), perhaps, in terms of *vicarious practise*. Similar to what Davie argued, itemised forms address religious affiliation and keep the necessary record to meet policy requirements and organisational guidelines as a hospice professional, and healthcare professional overall. Regardless of whether this is practised by all hospice professionals – whether they ask the questions and tick the boxes – these are practises that represent the vast majority of professionals in the field and who, according to this book's argument, agree with them. The itemised forms are both good and bad towards quality of care and religious literacy in hospice care. This is discussed in Chapter 8.

Neutral spaces

One of the proposed domains of quality of care refers to the hospice environment (Hospice UK, 2014). This was extensively discussed in Chapter 4 of this book. Yet, the practise of neutralizing space has further impact on professional practise.

The development and usage of neutral spaces in a hospice shows that religion and belief have been integrated in professional practise. This argument is further discussed by Pentaris and Thomsen (2018), who examined the various approaches in which hospice and palliative care is delivered in the UK and Denmark. Their study highlights the tendency to be neutral in order to respond to the diverse identities of service users; yet, this suggestion remains open to research and exploration.

This section suggests that hospice professionals demonstrate what Appleby (1999) described as religious misunderstandings. An increasing ambivalence towards engaging with religious diversity is evident, which perplexes the intentions of inclusive and holistic care. Of course, this is a somewhat expected reality. Vertovec (2010) discussed the changing context of diversity, putting emphasis on the new forms of migration and how those impact on host nations. In his exploration, Vertovec (2010) delves into an interpretive analysis of what is called post-multi-culturalism and how people engage with this concept. His analysis offered ideas of ambivalence towards the complexity of identity due to lack of understanding. Similarly, religious identity and belief have changed drastically in modern history (see Chapter 2), and such changes diversified individual identities even further, and naturally complicated the human experience related to religion, belief and spirituality. Box 7.4 contains some extracts, which highlight the meaning hospice professionals attach to neutral spaces.

Box 7.4

'We want to be neutral so that the hospice is friendly to all spiritualities' (Alex, age 44).

'This hospice is multi-faith, so in order to become very welcoming to all religions, we are neutral. There is no religious preference, and we try not to present religious signs often so that people of other groups are not offended' (John, age 53).

'We have got a spiritual care coordinator within our hospice, who facilitates our chaplaincy team, and therefore a variety of different religious denominations, and actually nonreligious denominations as well. We have a humanistic chaplain who deals with people who believe in something but don't actually pertain to any religious order as such' (Dorothy, age 37).

'Well, here it used to be an extremely Catholic institution and then it opened itself up, and it is now a very beautiful, holistic, and neutral space. And people around here have changed. They have understood that not everybody wants crucifixes and icons all around, so we have quiet rooms for prayers, etc. So, people have learned to be discreet with their religion too' (Anna, age 59).

Religious networking

The newly merged Network for Pastoral, Spiritual and Religious Care in Health (NPSRC) and the Chaplaincy Leadership Forum (CLF), now known as the *Healthcare Chaplaincy Forum for Pastoral, Spiritual and Religious Care*, underscored the significance of this aspect of care and the necessity for healthcare professionals to work together to ensure the care they deliver is effective and safe for the service users. In that, the Forum highlights the need for networking and expanding collaborations, for various reasons, including the ultimate purpose of meeting service user needs related to religion or belief.

The idea of multi-agency and interprofessional practise is not new, either in policy or in practise. Yet, the idea of religious networking has not long ago entered the discussion (e.g., Crawley et al., 2000) but has seen little progression since. There is relevance to organisational networking and inter-professional work. Hughes and Wearing (2017) suggest that effective professionalism is always benefitted by extensive and multi-skilled networks. This is to highlight the importance of involving all available professionals and skills towards working with the service user. An enhanced religious network serves a purpose but defeats another one, however. It enriches the experience of the service user by providing an additional service that seeks to promote further the care of the individual. On the other hand, it under-mines the capacity of hospice professionals to meet the service user needs, but through other practitioners. This may as well jeopardise the rapport that professionals build with service users, as the latter are referred to chaplains commonly after they request from a professional to be supported spiritually by them. In other words, service users request support by hospice profes-sionals, and instead they get a reference to the chaplain. Despite my argu-ment here, chaplaincies are very important in the care of service users in EOL and hospice care; nonetheless, disciplinary roles overlap and confuse different professionals. Also, chaplaincies are as well in need of 'becoming more religiously literate' (Gilliat-Ray and Clines, 2015, p. 237). Even though this book does not explore this at large, it makes recommendations that may generally apply to any professional involved in hospice care.

The positive impact of religious networking, as indicated earlier, is imper-ative and the role of chaplains, even though ambivalent by other disciplines (VandeCreek and Burton, 2001), complementary to the overall care of service users. Yet, there is still a dearth of data to support how religious networking in terms of referring service users to religious leaders is an appropriate or even sufficient response to needs related to religion, belief and spirituality overall. If we return to Chapter 3 of this book, it is apparent that policy endorses the role of chaplaincy in hospice care, but with little demonstration of what the role is specifically, under what circumstances and for whose benefit. The latter areas are just as opaque or clear as the definition or description of spiritual care (Hummel et al., 2009).

Box 7.5

'We have good and close relationships and collaboration with religious lead-ers and priests and other chapels in the community. So, they come in and provide services if necessary' (Janice, age 47).

'So, it is just recognising that it is like a bucket full of options that you can pick from and use different people at different times according to what is the highest need at the time. So, spiritual care comprises from a whole range of people – chaplains, sometimes the imam, sometimes it is the holy man, whomever – but we have got a range of people to meet the range of people we provide service for' (Anna, age 59).

'You respect all people's beliefs, and support them ... what they need in their final days, and how to cope with the dying process, and that is fine. And one of the good things about this place is, you name your own religion, we will have somebody available for it. Yes, we have a rabbi who comes visits, we have an imam, who is available to be called on, we have a Catholic priest, we have got a Church of England, and when we need somebody from any religion ... we just call someone' (Carol, age 42).

Hospice professionals appear to rely heavily on religious networks to promote spiritual care, inclusive of religion and belief, as well as nonreli-gion and nonbelief. Despite the positive aspects of this approach, which are seen in detail in Nolan (2011), this book contests the efficiency of this method on the whole. Religion, belief and spiritual needs are either per-ceived as itemised, outcome-measured aspects of care or a conceptual and phenomenologically understood human experience. Processing requests through referral systems and relying on the capacity of a religious network of a hospice may suggest that the service user's needs are experienced on a more practical level (discussed in Chapter 6). This book's overall argument, though, lies in the roots of how religion, belief and spirituality – inclusive of nonreligion or nonbelief – as human experience are integrated in hospice care specifically and end of life care generally.

To extend this discussion and highlight how hospice professionals may exemplify the integration of such identities in practise, Box 7.5 offers some extracts which not only demonstrate my claim, but also stress the contro-versy in it: Professionals are open to offering support around the domain of spirituality and religion, but religious networking is how religion, belief and spirituality are integrated in professional practise.

Commemorative practises

A final but important area to tackle is that of *commemorative practises* – in other words, supportive acts during one's dying or following a bereave-ment. This area reflects an overlap of religion, tradition and ritual (also see

Arfman, 2014); yet, hospice professionals appreciate such acts as a reflection of how religion, belief and spirituality are integrated in practise.

Initially, we need to examine and critically approach the functional roles of rituals before we link them to religion and supportive acts in hospice care. Cultural anthropology has offered that the overall role of rituals is that they promote a peaceful death, as well as bring reconciliation and acceptance to the bereaved and the dying. Last, rituals act as links between an earthly presence and a higher power – human nature and divine presence. These are reflected in the following paragraphs, which explore the work of Van Gennep (2011) and Turner (1967, 1977, 1979).

Van Gennep (2011) suggests that rites of passage accompany all changes in life, and that people's stories are crowded with passages from one life situation to another. Van Gennep identifies three phases that mark all rites of passage and rituals. Those phases are separation, margin (or limen, meaning 'threshold' in Latin), and aggregation. The first phase signifies detachment from one fixed point in a past social structure, followed by a form of symbolic behaviour. The second is the intervening period during which individuals pass through unfamiliar elements. Third, during aggregation, the passage is consummated and individuals find themselves in a stable state once more. With these three phases in mind, commemorative practises in hospice care offer service users the opportunity to process their experience and grow from it.

Turner (1967), on the other hand, observes four phases in the processional form of rituals: breach of regular norm, crisis or extension of the breach, readdressive or adjusting mechanisms, and reintegration of the disturbed social group. This was what he called the 'social drama' (Social drama has been introduced as a device to look carefully underneath the surface of social regulations and norms and into contradictions and controversies within society.) Turner (1967, p. 19) defined ritual as a 'prescribed formal behaviour for occasions not given to technological routine, having reference to beliefs in mystical beings and powers'. He further opines that 'the ritual system compensates to some extent for the limited range of effective political control and for the instability of kinship and affiance ties to which political value is attached' (p. 291). Drawing on these descriptors, commemorative practises, which often materialise through ritual, seem to respond to the structure of hospice care through a more relaxed and accommodating manner, whilst taking into account beliefs and traditions – religious or not – which are not otherwise considered.

Another definition of Turner's (1967, p. 183) is that ritual is 'a stereotyped sequence of activities involving gestures, words, and objects, performed in a sequestered place, and designed to influence preternatural entities or forces on behalf of the actors' goals and interests'. This definition encompasses the diversity of means by which rituals materialise, as well as highlights their recurrent nature.

Following on from this descriptor, rituals are comprised of symbols, and symbols, more often than not, present social and religious values – often overlapping.

Turner (1977) distinguished between *dominant* and *instrumental* symbols. Dominant symbols appear in many ritual contexts, but their meaning comprises a high level of autonomy and consistency in the symbolic system. Instrumental symbols, though, are the means of attaining specific goals of ritual performance. The separation of symbols not only reflects the different ways in which they are used in rituals, but also helps us appreciate the varied implications of the use of symbols in commemorative practises.

Furthermore, Turner's (1979) processual view on rituals is informed by Van Gennep's analysis of rites of passage (1909 [1960]). Turner suggests that ritual is situated within a process of social drama and is processual in form. The processual view of rituals is presented with a distinction between life-crisis rituals (these mark a transition in a person's life, from one developmental point to the next) and rituals of affliction (rituals performed for individuals who are 'caught' by the spirit of the lost one) (Turner, 1967).

Also, Turner (1967) separated the field in which rituals take place; he identified the social and cultural fields. The former refers to societal principles and groups and relationships in which rituals are performed, whereas the latter considers ritual symbols that represent meaning. These two fields reflect the aforementioned argument of Turner's that wants rituals to present social and religious values. With further examination, Turner defines rituals as acts inclusive of religion as practise, and belief as religious thought.

A last note that is worthy of attention is *communitas*. Turner (1967) used the term to describe that all ritual subjects in the liminal phase in the ritual process are treated equally, free from characteristics of social structure. This view on ritual has been adopted by Van Gennep's (2011) work as well, whilst it informs our understanding of commemorative practises, which is the aim of this section.

Hospice professionals express wider acceptance of commemorative practises, such as holding ceremonies, sending cards and creating memory books, as an established form of how religion, belief and spirituality are integrated in practise (Box 7.6). This is not far from Turner's and Van Gennep's observations and suggestions, in which both identify the links between rituals, symbols and religion or belief.

Scholars around hospice practise, religion and death, more generally, have identified these but from different angles. Walter (2003) explored the

---

Box 7.6

'A ceremony – light up a life – which is a commemorative ceremony where the death of somebody is remembered and respected, and the light is to represent their life. We have many of those practises, like adding people's names on the metal leaves to remember them' (Margarita, age 36).

'There are memory books with names and the opportunity for people to write how they feel in commemoration. That might include a lot of feelings because of their religion' (Mirna, age 48).

role of chaplains in the process of providing rites after death and in the year to come in hospice care. In his work, he found that such rites are indeed beneficial to service users, yet not all hospices engage with such activities; some find these rites to be morbid. Similarly, Macdonald et al. (2005) found that bereaved individuals – specifically parents – appreciated commemorative practises in general, and as a platform from which to express personal values and beliefs specifically. When such supportive acts were lacking, it was noticed, emphasising the importance of carrying them out. Another equal example is the noted in the work by Davies et al. (2007) which highlights the benefits of commemorative practises and its links to values and beliefs, whether religious or spiritual.

Despite the benefits from commemorative practises, there seems to be some discrepancy regarding people for whom religion or belief are important, and their counterparts. Commemoration of the deceased as evidence of accommodating belief, in other words, seems to focus on religion and traditional practises; however, there are secular and nonreligious beliefs that may not fit this approach.

Concluding thoughts

This chapter portrayed hospice professionals' identification of five ways in which religion, belief and spirituality are integrated in practise: policy, assessment, neutrality of the space, religious networking and commemorative practises. It is now worth returning to Puchalski's (2007–2008) typology of spiritual care and contrasting it with these five approaches in practise.

To revisit the typology, Puchalski (2007–2008) explains that the intrinsic aspect of care refers to compassionate care whereas extrinsic is the aspect that describes more practical ways in which religion-, belief- and spiritual-related needs are addressed. The first impression, from looking at all five approaches/practises discussed in this chapter, is that they belong to the extrinsic aspect of spiritual care. Policy presents guidelines for practise but rarely specifies how the guidelines are to materialise. Also, the guidelines are either explicit, to meet practical needs, or more generic – for example, to meet spiritual needs – and are open to interpretation, but with little demand for a compassionate presence. Equally, the practise of gathering information during an initial assessment lacks depth to allow the professional to appreciate and understand how the service connects with service users' identity and how to make sense of it. It does, however, allow professionals to address more practical issues later, such as dietary requirements. On the same note, promoting neutrality in the space enables individuals to address practical issues, such as misunderstandings from people with a faith not represented in the space. Religious networking is an interesting approach as it highlights the tendency to refer people elsewhere to have their needs met. Even though religious leaders represent, in their role, much more of the compassionate presence described with intrinsic care (also see Nolan, 2011), service users notice the lack of engagement from the hospice professionals' perspective. Commemorative practises are an ambiguous approach. On the one hand, such practises offer space for meeting practical needs (e.g., signing a memory book, as is the tradition in the deceased's faith), but on the other, they become means of compassionate presence even if the hospice professional is not present.

Drawing on this contrast – between how professionals respond to religion, belief and spiritual identities, and the intrinsic and extrinsic aspects of spiritual care – it is inevitable that one may question the approaches identified in this chapter. This is not because they do not, indeed, meet some needs, but because they are lacking in amplitude – in other words, the capacity to engage adequately with service users' identities related to their belief system, to begin both to understand and appreciate the meaning of this system for the individual and how it impacts on their perception of their experience.

A determining question, then, is how far are these approaches and ways in which professionals find comfort in responding to the needs of the service users practise models. Equally important is the question of how much of the practise is a coping strategy. I have elsewhere (Pentaris, 2018) argued that hospice professionals, like nurses, social workers and physicians, do not always present themselves as comfortable with this task. Often, due to inability or lack of understanding, professionals find ways to cope with the ambiguous and challenging task of meeting such needs. An example is making spaces neutral. It is questionable how much this attitude accommodates people's needs, rather than masking inclusivity for neutrality, which ultimately satisfies organisational and policy needs.

This chapter does not provide answers to the questions in the preceding paragraph, yet stirs the conversation further and draws readers' attention to the need for exploring the binary of coping strategies and practise models to have a clearer picture of how religion, belief and spiritual identities are treated in hospice practise.

References

Alcock, P., 2014. *Social policy in Britain*. London: Palgrave Macmillan.

Appleby, S.R., 1999. *The ambivalence of the sacred: Religion, violence, and reconciliation*. London, UK: Rowman & Littlefield.

Arfman, W., 2014. Innovating from traditions: The emergence of a ritual field of collective commemoration in the Netherlands. *Journal of Contemporary Religion*, 29(1), pp. 17–32.

Catto, R. and Perfect, D., 2015. Religious literacy, equalities and human rights. In Dinham, A. and Francis, M. (eds.), *Religious literacy in policy and practice*. Bristol: Policy Press, pp. 135–163.

Crawley, L., Payne, R., Bolden, J., Payne, T., Washington, P. and Williams, S., 2000. Palliative and end-of-life care in the African American community. *Journal of the American Medical Association*, 284(19), pp. 2518–2521.

Daaleman, T.P., Usher, B.M., Williams, S.W., Rawlings, J. and Hanson, L.C., 2008. An exploratory study of spiritual care at the end of life. *The Annals of Family Medicine*, 6(5), pp. 406–411.

Davie, G., 2013. *The sociology of religion: A critical agenda*. London, UK: Sage.

Davie, G., 2007. Vicarious religion: A methodological challenge. In Ammerman, N.T. (ed.), *Everyday religion: Observing modern religious lives*. New York, NY: Oxford University Press, pp. 21–36.

Davies, B., Collins, J., Steele, R. and Cook, K., 2007. Parents' and children's perspectives of a children's hospice bereavement program. *Journal of Palliative Care*, 23(1), pp. 14–23.

Furman, L.D., Benson, P.W., Grimwood, C. and Canda, E., 2004. Religion and spirituality in social work education and direct practice at the millennium: A survey of UK social workers. *British Journal of Social Work*, 34(6), pp. 767–792.

Gilliat-Ray, S. and Clines, J., 2015. Religious literacy and chaplaincy. In Dinham, A. and Francis, M. (eds.), *Religious literacy in policy and practice*. Bristol: Policy Press, pp. 237–256.

Hospice UK, 2014. *Defining quality in hospice care*. London, UK: Hospice UK. Available at: https://www.hospiceuk.org/docs/default-source/default-document-library/defining-quality-in-hospice-care.pdf?sfvrsn=4.

Hughes, M. and Wearing, M., 2017. *Organisations and management in social work: Everyday action for change*. London, UK: Sage.

Hummel, L., Galek, K., Murphy, K.M., Tannenbaum, H.P. and Flannelly, L.T., 2009. Defining spiritual care: An exploratory study. *Journal of Health Care Chaplaincy*, 15(1), pp. 40–51.

James, N. and Field, D., 1992. The routinization of hospice: Charisma and bureaucratization. *Social Science & Medicine*, 34(12), pp. 1363–1375.

Macdonald, M.E., Liben, S., Carnevale, F.A., Rennick, J.E., Wolf, S.L., Meloche, D. and Cohen, S.R., 2005. Parental perspectives on hospital staff members' acts of kindness and commemoration after a child's death. *Pediatrics*, 116(4), pp. 884–890.

Nolan, S., 2011. *Spiritual care at the end of life: The chaplain as a 'hopeful presence'*. London, UK: Jessica Kingsley.

Pentaris, P., 2018. The marginalisation of religion in end of life care: Signs of microaggression? *International Journal of Human Rights in Healthcare*, 11(2), pp. 116–128.

Pentaris, P., 2014. Religion, secularism, and professional practice. *STUDIA Sociologica-Annales Universitatis Paedagogicae Cracoviensis*, 6(1), pp. 99–109.

Pentaris, P. and Thomsen, L.L., 2018. Cultural and religious diversity in hospice and palliative care: A qualitative cross-country comparative analysis of the challenges of healthcare professionals. *Omega: Journal of Death and Dying,* Accepted paper.

Phillips, J.L. and Agar, M.R., 2016. Exemplary nursing leadership is central to improving care of the dying. *Journal of Nursing Management*, 24(1), pp. 1–3.

Puchalski, C.M., 2007–2008. Spirituality and the care of patients at the end-of-life: An essential component of care. *Omega: Journal of Death and Dying*, 56(1), pp. 33–46.

Reese, D.J., Melton, E. and Ciaravino, K., 2004. Programmatic barriers to providing culturally competent end-of-life care. *American Journal of Hospice and Palliative Medicine*, 21(5), pp. 357–364.

Tan, S.Y., 1996. Religion in clinical practice: Implicit and explicit integration. In Shafranske, E. (ed.), *Religion and the clinical practice of psychology*. Washington, DC: American Psychological Association, pp. 365–390.

Turner, V., 1979. Dramatic ritual/ritual drama: Performative and reflexive anthropology. *The Kenyon Review*, 1(3), pp. 80–93.

Turner, V., 1977. Variations on a theme of liminality. In Moore, S.F. and Myerhoff, B.G. (eds.), *Secular ritual*. Assen: Gorcum, pp. 36–52.

Turner, V.W., 1967. *The forest of symbols: Aspects of Ndembu ritual*, vol. 101. Ithaca, NY: Cornell University Press.

VandeCreek, L. and Burton, L. (eds.), 2001. Professional chaplaincy: Its role and importance in healthcare. *Journal of Pastoral Care & Counseling*, 55(1), pp. 81–97.

Van Gennep, A., 2011. *The rites of passage*. Chicago: University of Chicago Press.

Van Gennep, A., 1960. *The rites of passage*. (Vizedom, M.B. and Caffee, G.L., trans.). Chicago: University of Chicago Press.

Vertovec, S., 2010. Towards post-multiculturalism? Changing communities, conditions and contexts of diversity. *International Social Science Journal*, 61(199), pp. 83–95.

Walter, T., 2003. Hospices and rituals after death: A survey of British hospice chaplains. *International Journal of Palliative Nursing*, 9(2), pp. 80–85.

Wolf, C.T. and Stevens, P., 2001. Integrating religion and spirituality in marriage and family counseling. *Counseling and Values*, 46(1), pp. 66–75.

Young, C.S. and Young, J.S., 2014. *Integrating spirituality and religion into counseling: A guide to competent practice*. London, UK: Wiley.

Zimmermann, C., 2012. Acceptance of dying: A discourse analysis of palliative care literature. *Social Science & Medicine*, 75(1), pp. 217–224.

Part III

Religious literacy in hospice care

8 Religious literacy in hospice care

Introduction

Hospice professionals are undeniably willing to engage with the religion, belief and spiritual identities of service users, but may often lack the appropriate language and skills to do so. This book underlines that, in general, professionals always act in the best interest of service users, but with limitations about which they may be unaware. In other words, the level of religious literacy in end of life care in general, and hospice care specifically, seems dubious. This ambiguity is evidence in support of a few of the conclusions discussed later in this chapter.

This book highlights a current trend among professionals in EOL care: the perception that knowing more about more religions will result in religious literacy or will otherwise better prepare professionals to work with people from different religious backgrounds. However, this is not a proven fact. As suggested by Dinham and Francis (2015), religious literacy is not about knowing it all. Religious literacy, at least in hospice care, and as it has been used in this volume as a theoretical approach, is a process related to interpersonal skills. It is also a process for minimizing and managing ambivalence towards difference. The lack of engagement – at least on an intrinsic level – with religion, belief and spiritual identities might also be due to feelings of unease. Hospice staff may feel intimidated by difference more broadly, not necessarily just by religious differences. This is, of course, a hypothesis to be examined in a different project, yet it is worth noting. This assumption is also supported by the following: In hospice care, a Christian-centred approach is often employed and professionals show more and better quality engagement when the service user is of Christian belief or background.

As discussed in Chapter 1, EOL care is highly contextualised. Death, dying and bereavement are unparalleled experiences which deserve absolute and comprehensive attention. In the UK, by and large, EOL care is practised in hospices, fitting into the concept of palliative care. That said, EOL care is often guided by bio-medical approaches, and clinical and legal frameworks, and these are frequently far from psychosocial and interpersonal assessments and interventions. It is rather enticing to ask whether hospice care has turned into hospice cure. Aside from the arguments around this question, it is clear that religion and belief remain marginalised from professional practise unless they are regarded as problems to be solved (Pentaris, 2018a).

Religion, belief and spirituality are integral aspects of individuals' identity, or intrinsic to their identity as a whole. They are also aspects that do not exist in a static form; neither do they have a descriptive character. In other words, these are lived experiences that can be understood through actions and behaviours. According to Dollard (1983, p. 7), 'one simple way of understanding spirituality is to see that it is concerned with our ability, through our attitudes and actions, to relate to others, to ourselves, and to God as we understand Him'. Dame Cicely Saunders saw this when setting up hospice care, and so did many others after her. Nevertheless, as the bio-medical and clinical models took hold, hospice care became crowded with policies and regulations that were at times influenced by political ideologies and which naturally led to radical changes in the organisational foundations – if we are treating hospice care as an organisation. Over the course of time, hospice care was filled with professionals willing to engage with multiple aspects of care, but with limited or no proper language – and therefore no skills (Furness and Gilligan, 2010) – to do so in some areas (also see Pentaris, 2018a).

This book explored the challenges and controversies that hospice professionals face when required to engage with the religious beliefs, nonreligious values and spiritual identities of service users. It transpires from the second part of the book that professionals are willing to engage with these aspects of care, but nonetheless lack the religious literacy to address them adequately and sensitively. Chapter 3 delved into social policy and how religion and belief are played out in these fields. It was noted, neither exhaustively nor comprehensively, that muddled and inconsistent guidelines cause distress and controversies within professional practise situations, such as itemised forms. In this chapter, I highlight the most fundamental outcomes of this book and the research project (Pentaris, 2016) underpinning its arguments. However, before I do so, it is important to discuss briefly the context and generalised issues regarding this book, and how they influence the applicability of the religious literacy for hospice care model proposed later in the chapter.

EOL has a wide context. There are various settings in which people live at EOL – hospice, care home, hospital or in their own home, to name a few. This variety may as well suggest a variety of approaches and attitudes towards religion, belief and spirituality in EOL care overall, based on the setting in which it is explored. This is an important recognition as it influences the generalisability of the arguments offered in this book.

Pentaris (2016) has explored religious literacy in hospice care, which limits the application of the findings across other settings within the overall landscape of EOL care. However, this book draws on perspectives and attitudes from a varied sample of hospice professionals who may also be practising in the community or other than hospice settings (e.g., care homes).

The conversation about spirituality is not an unwelcome one in a hospice – a setting that seems to provide conventional healthcare. Nevertheless, hospice professionals appear uncomfortable discussing religion and belief. This may be partially because of the institutionalised care setting in which my study (Pentaris, 2016) was undertaken. Perhaps in the community there is more freedom of discussion about religion and belief. When people near the end of their lives are cared for in their own home, separate rules may apply about what is acceptable or welcoming as a subject for a conversation. An example of this is seen in Owens and Randhawa (2004). They examined community-based palliative care of South Asian people in the UK. In their account, they argue that a community-based model enhances the opportunity for more culturally competent care, inclusive of religion, as service users feel restricted in the institutional setting of hospice services. However, the identified contrast between in-patient and community-based hospice care in relation to spiritual care (inclusive of religion and belief) does not necessitate that the latter is not challenged in community-based practise. Luker et al. (2000) identified some of the challenges pertaining to community nursing of terminally ill patients. Their study concluded that the major challenge nurses face is to ensure a strong and meaningful relationship with patients to get to know them better and, hence, offer higher quality spiritual care.

Two of the fundamental findings of my study (Pentaris, 2016), explored later in this section, are the general ambivalence towards religion and belief and the tendency to treat religious diversification as a problem that requires appropriate solutions. Both are key to understanding how religion, belief and spirituality are perceived in and embedded into hospice care, or healthcare in general (also see Cobb, Puchalski and Rumbold, 2012). As discussed earlier, this may not be as representative of service provision in the community. Perhaps hospice professionals in the community overcome their ambivalence to approaching this subject with service users because policies inform practise differently in that area (see Chapter 3). Similarly, hospice professionals may show more religious literacy when working in the community, and as a result engage with that aspect of the service user's identity whilst avoiding treating it as problematic or contradictory to the bio-medical culture evident in hospice and palliative care (Nebel Pederson and Emmers-Sommer, 2012). Religious belief and practise commonly take place in the community in an everyday context (McGuire, 2008), and service users may already find support and promotion of their religious and spiritual wellbeing there. Professionals may not consider spiritual care a priority when working in the community, yet ought to appreciate the difference between professional and personal perspectives of care, and complement the support individuals receive from their social and communal circles.

Service users in hospices receive holistic care that addresses all their identified needs. Social policy recognises the responsibility of hospice professionals to meet the spiritual needs of service users in hospice care, but not necessarily those of service users encountered when working in the community (Department of Health, 2008). This makes the research question about how religion, belief and spirituality are integrated in practise even more pressing. If policies highlight such a responsibility within institutional care, then logic requires that professionals be adequately prepared for this task, however ambiguous.

This introduction briefly touches on various challenging circumstances observed in current hospice care and the way in which religion, belief and spirituality are negotiated within them. The next few sections extensively discuss the main challenges identified and also highlight the controversies that accompany them.

Religious literacy in hospice care

The following sections highlight and discuss the themes emerging from the second part of this book. Each section tackles one recurrent theme, but all interconnect and should be read as one account.

Secular hospice or hospice with its religious fur cast off

The origins of contemporary hospice care are strongly religious – Christian, to be specific. The Hospices de Beaune in 15th-century France were structured and led by Christian beliefs, and their interior architecture more closely resembled that of a church than a hospice or hospital for the poor. Equally, the Dames de Calaire institution, founded by Madame Jeanne Garnier in Lyon in 1842, was led by Madame Garnier's religious beliefs and founded on those principles. More generally, the history of the term 'hospice' is itself religious. It has been used since the fourth century to refer to the care of the sick and the dying as defined by Christian orders and denominations. In other words, hospice care is intrinsically connected with Christianity.

In many ways, hospice care continues to retain its religious identity even now. Its historically religious values and ideals are evidently informing contemporary practise on organisational and foundational levels. Indeed, despite the development and evolvement of hospices that affirm a nonreligious, all-religions-inclusive, or neutral identity, foundational norms and practises are embedded in religious values, which are institutionalised within hospice care. Therefore, it is possible to argue that modern hospice care provides a form of secular care, but without separating religious norms and values from the organisational and foundational status (also see Campbell, 2012). Also, in response to changes in religious practise and belief (discussed in Chapter 2), hospices have been challenged and made certain adjustments to respond to the increasingly diverse religion and belief environment. Some of these adjustments are more practical (e.g., removing religious items from hospice walls) and others are more conceptual (e.g., recommendations to professionals to refrain from delving into actions pertaining to religion or belief).

Not unlike the various initiatives in modern history (e.g., migrant health policies [see Mladovsky et al., 2012]), which respond to diversity in societies, hospices appear to consider diversity in religion as a problem to be solved. Furthermore, hospice care's solutions need to be responsive to equality and diversity laws and procedures (e.g., Equality Act 2010). Alternatively, instead of treating the new environment as a multi-faith and diverse context, it is often seen as a Christian context which now needs to accommodate other identities as well. This is reflective of the need for cultural humility (Hook et al., 2013), which needs practise to break free of normative and conventional behaviours and embrace a lack of superiority in order to be inclusive and unbiased.

In an effort to be inclusive and non-judgemental, as well as to avoid tension among different religious groups, hospices now project themselves as more neutral spaces. From the arguments in this book, it is clear that the hospice space has become less and less religious. Icons and crucifixes are removed, religious signs are withdrawn and the language on signs is changed – all these with few exceptions. Is this space secular? Or does it remain religious – Christian – but hides its religiousness in the name of inclusivity? I am, under no circumstances, suggesting that hospice care should not be an all-inclusive system of care. Rather, I am contesting the way this is realised – masking inclusivity with neutrality. Religious foundations in hospices remain pertinent to hospice care nowadays. However, hospices are faced with the challenge of balancing their religious history and foundations with the more current and contemporary social construct of religious, nonreligious or spiritual identity.

The neutrality of hospice space gives rise to an additional dialogue. Dinham and Francis (2015) note that *secular* is often regarded as *neutral* and vice versa. This book was not concerned with examining this argument in depth, but rather concludes that hospices are either in the process of secularising *or* they are ensuring that anything related to religion is removed from the public spaces within the organisation. Regardless, the lack of presence of religious items in the spaces of a hospice further supports the argument that there is a lack of religious literacy in hospice care, as this book shows with empirical findings. This is not to undermine the positive developments in hospice care, but to highlight that there is still a lot of ground to cover towards religiously literate professional practise – or, as I prefer to think about it, *humane practise*.

Religious belief and practise in neutral spaces

Service users are still in need of a space where they are comfortable to pray or find 'peace of mind'. Chapels have changed radically and the use of prayer rooms has become popular in public institutions. As previous chapters describe, prayer rooms have been transformed into quiet rooms to promote equality and inclusivity. Gilliat-Ray (2005, p. 288) suggested that space for worship is necessary and that institutions should 'create rooms that can be used by people of "all faiths, or none"'. Hence, quiet rooms. The removal of the word *prayer* widens the space for all religions or none. Yet, how far a quiet room, instead of a prayer room, welcomes or represents people who identify with religion is still to be answered.

The findings of this study suggest that hospice service users do not make the expected use of quiet rooms, although there are exceptions. During the period of participant observation in the hospice, service users only made use of the quiet room when family members and friends were visiting an in-patient. On those occasions, the quiet room served as a lounge, a space for social interactions and perhaps more private conversations. Nevertheless, service users still look for an appropriate space for prayers or spiritual comfort. This is evident in the finding that service users make use of the garden to find peace and pray. This gives rise to the hypothesis that quiet rooms are not used as one would expect them to be.

The conclusion drawn from this book is that people with religious beliefs still find themselves lacking an appropriate space to express their beliefs and values. From quiet rooms, we now find service users retreating to the garden as a temple of peace and worship – a place for prayers and believing. This finding informs us in terms of service user needs and further illuminates whether, and to what extent, professional practise meets service user needs.

Willingness versus ability

One of the most fundamental outcomes of this book is concerned with the ability, as opposed to the willingness, of hospice professionals to talk about and engage with the religion, belief and spiritual identities of service users. As noted by Dinham and Francis (2015, p. 5), 'the problem is not people's willingness to have the conversations; it is their ability to do so'.

Chapter 2 went into detailed discussion of the new and changing religious landscape in the UK, together with the challenges society faces regarding the way in which religion and belief are treated publicly. Religion and belief are now considered absent from public life, with the discourse on secularisation increasing. Post-war Britain saw many developments and transformations in the nation, one of which was that of the composition of its population. The country publicly identified with its radically diversifying environment, and many and varied religious beliefs found a place, with solutions being sought for accommodation of these diverse identities. In this space, however, secularity took hold in conversation, whereas the decline in religious practise was seen as a decline in belief. As explored in the second chapter, the changing religious landscape in the post-war years, the change of language (i.e., from religious to secular) within the welfare state, as well as the lack of common understanding of contested notions, such as belief and faith, have all led to people losing their ability to talk about religion and belief when necessary.

Religion became a private matter with limited attention given to it in the public sphere. Consequentially, the ability to address this issue properly in policy, practise or education faded. Concurrently, in health and social care, bio-medical and clinical approaches took hold, at the expense of the psychosocial and the spiritual, the latter being absorbed into the psychosocial (discussed in the preceding chapters). Spiritual care became integral to hospice care and got more publicity in the late 20th century (McSherry, 2001). Spirituality was now used as a proxy for religion and belief. The thesis of this book has not been concerned with the distinction between the two (if there is one). Rather, it suggests that religion, belief and spirituality should be seen as relevant to the unique lived experiences of an individual. They may be momentous in terms of perceptions and meaning-making in life (also explored in Chapter 1); death and dying are often experienced through the lens of belief or faith, religious or not.

It is essential that hospice professionals who support people towards the end of their lives, or those who are grieving, have the ability to engage properly and address needs relating to religion, belief and spirituality together with the person's experience of dying and/or grieving. Religious literacy in hospice care, as well as EOL care in general, does not refer to a 'know-it-all' attitude in terms of learning more about many different religious traditions or denominations. The latter was indicated in interviewees' responses (Chapters 5 and 6), in which all participants suggested in various ways that they seize opportunities to learn practical information about different religions. Professionals do so to avoid *acting surprised* when they work with a service user from a religious tradition unfamiliar to them. In Pentaris (2016), hospice professionals suggested that being aware of something also makes them prepared to respond to it. This leads us to think that hospice professionals lack appreciation of the general sensitivity with which difference between people is treated. Religious literacy is not concerned with any of this, but with the ability to ask appropriate questions when needed, as well as the ability to engage comfortably with the subject as necessary.

> It is obvious that nobody can know everything about every religion and belief, and religions and beliefs are not homogeneous slabs of knowable 'stuff' in any case. The reality is of religion and belief as shifting aspects of contested identity. But engagement in the detail and the reality of at least some religion and belief, and an ability to ask appropriate questions with confidence about others, is an essential part of the journey. (Dinham and Francis, 2015, p. 14)

The findings of Pentaris (2016) lead to two possible scenarios. First, that professionals in hospice care have an inaccurate perception of what is beneficial and efficient in terms of responding to religion, belief and spiritual identities. This perception is perhaps the result of secular-minded education in health and social care professions, which prepare professionals to perform efficiently and sufficiently in a secular context. There is a general perception that acquisition of further knowledge about more and various religions will lead to the desired outcome: sensitive professional practise when it comes to the personal characteristics of service users and their family members or friends. Hospice professionals appear to consider that having knowledge of religious practises and traditions equates to having the abilities and skills to work sensitively in a multi-faith environment. This book contests this idea and suggests that religious literacy goes beyond that and is necessary to perceive the duty of professional practise more clearly in conjunction with the ongoing changes and needs of service users.

The second scenario suggests that hospice organisations lead professionals to develop secular-minded perceptions about working within a multi-faith environment, or sustain the secular perceptions gained in their education or training. This is highly challenging as it contradicts organisational foundations and the roots of hospice care (see Chapter 1). Equally, this book contests this approach to practise, from an organisational perspective, and suggests that hospice settings can further diversify professionals' practise and the way skills and knowledge are communicated to them. It seems imperative to find a perfect balance between organisational foundations, organisational culture, health and social care professions' education, and training and service user needs.

Ambivalence

Lack of proper abilities to engage well with religion, belief and spirituality has led hospice professionals to become ambivalent towards talking about religion and belief. Professionals who participated in this study expressed the opinion that they do not wish to talk about religion and belief for various reasons, including guidance from an organisational perspective. As is reported in Chapters 5 and 6, professionals choose to use the term 'spirituality' when engaging in a conversation about religious and nonreligious beliefs. It is presented as almost a taboo, for example, to talk about Judaism or Hinduism.

Professionals in hospices appear to be fairly ambivalent towards the subject of religion, and most of their reasons for this hinge upon the concepts of equality and diversity. Lack of engagement seems to be rationalised by employing neutral behaviours and attitudes that accommodate all differences within the service user composition. Such approaches, however, seem counterproductive – avoiding identifying and engaging with diversity to accommodate diverse identities. This is reminiscent of Watson's (2015) work about secular ideas and the privatisation of religion. Watson (2015) identifies some inconsistencies in the secularist organisation of society, one of which suggests that the claim of neutral societies is dubious.

> [The] claim to *neutrality* may be bogus. It tends to be assumed that not mentioning something makes for neutrality when it can easily

lead to reductionism. Not mentioning God in the public domain may constitute practical atheism whether stated or not. It can convey the implication that religion is peripheral to the conduct of human affairs and therefore irrelevant. This is not any less contentious than the various religious views a secularist approach wishes to confine to the private sphere. Thus, built into the use of the term is a commitment to a controversial view of the world. That is not a neutral position. (Watson, 2015, p. 1458)

When considering the wider picture of how spiritual care occurs in hospices, the most tangible evidence is a set of questions professionals ask servicer users during their initial assessment. This book affirms that hospice professionals may consider practises analogous to the one mentioned earlier (see Chapter 6); proof of religious literacy in hospice care. In addition, professionals assert that their practise is necessarily informed by national and organisational policies and guidelines. When asked specifically how they engage with religion and belief, professionals suggest that asking service users about their faith when they are admitted is what organisational policies and recommendations suggest. This is problematic in that it supports the conclusion of ambivalence. It also suggests that if policies and guidelines (mostly equality and diversity laws) did not require hospice staff members to ask service users these questions, they might not do so. There is a mix of willingness to engage, ambivalence towards difference, lack of appropriate language to interconnect, and a need to follow the rules as the technocratic culture of hospice care suggests. This makes for a much more complicated context, in which ambivalence is one aspect alone.

Finding solutions

Equally important is the way in which religious diversity is perceived in hospice care. A very common theme that emerged from the discussion earlier in Chapters 6 and 7 is a solution-focused approach when addressing religious or nonreligious identities. This approach is observed in Dinham's and Francis's account (2015) in terms of how religion and belief are treated in different parts of public life.

> [I]t would be much more effective – and much more realistic – to set religion and belief in their proper context as normal, mainstream and widespread, and to seek engagement *with* them rather than solution *for* them. (Dinham and Francis 2015, p. 7)

Pentaris and Thomsen (2018) asserted that palliative and hospice care professionals in the UK and Denmark often approach both culture and faith, in their diversity, from a solutions-focussed perspective. Although this is not the stated aim, the authors drew on their comparative analysis to conclude that practise is becoming more and more concerned with factual knowledge and how that facilitates the process of 'finding solutions for emerging issues' – one being diversity.

The urge to find solutions seems to be an unforeseen consequence of a care system led by the principles of inclusivity, interpersonal communication and patient engagement. In such care systems, service user characteristics are often determined to be elements that prevent service delivery from being efficient. It almost appears as if hospice care, instead of accommodating diverse identities, attempts to find ways (i.e., solutions) to respond to the challenge of multiple religion-, belief- and spirituality-related identities. This endeavour in hospice care, though, puts the emphasis on the service and not the service user. A distinctive example of this is evidenced in Chapter 6, where hospice professionals respond to service user requests in relation to religion, belief and spirituality with a phone call to the chaplaincy team – or any other form of referral. This response seems rather dismissive and perhaps somewhat coloured with a 'quick fix' attitude.

In their narrative on religious literacy and chaplaincies, Clines with Gilliat-Ray (2015, p. 237) suggest that 'developing religious literacy within the chaplaincy and collaborating with others in an organization ... can be responsive to the breadth of religion and belief identities of its constituents'. The findings in Pentaris (2016) are far from suggesting that this is the attitude employed by professionals in hospice care (i.e., collaboration). On the contrary, what is shown is that hospice staff do not directly engage with the religious or nonreligious identities of service users unless on a pragmatic level. An example of this includes signposting service users to the chaplaincy team, with which there is little connection or collaboration (for communication and collaboration across and within human service organisations, see Hughes and Wearing [2017]).

In addition, hospice care currently projects and endorses the opinion that knowing about a service user's religion, belief or spiritual identity is not beneficial unless there are practical ways to accommodate such identities. For example, if a patient is Muslim, hospice professionals prepare to assist the patient in being able to die in a way appropriate to the teachings of Islam, as is supported in hospice settings. Again, this is problematic and only supports the finding of a problem-solving attitude rather than one that leads to a better understanding of how people comprehend their beliefs and what they mean to them, as well as how those beliefs inform their experience. Also, it suggests that professionals often retreat to pragmatic and general practise which will safeguard their professionalism, rather than reaching into the realms of intangible and unmeasurable care. This can be linked with the third chapter of this book and the discussion about how policy and legislation influence practise: the UK government's response to the review of choice in EOL care (i.e., *Our Commitment to You for End of Life Care – 2016* [Department of Health, 2016]) highlighted the need for highly coordinated and measured care to regulate properly choice in EOL care. This is one of many examples which show the tendency to continue this achievement-based and measurement-focussed drive on organisational and national levels.

The previous example also conceals a risk: generalising. Remember that Day's work (2009, 2011), found that being affiliated with one religion means no more than that; belief is not measured by affiliation or religious practise. Professionals in Pentaris (2016) did not address different religions in terms of different ways of believing or different beliefs. On the contrary, my study (Pentaris, 2016) suggests that hospice professionals tend to generalise their knowledge about one religious tradition across all service users who affiliate with it. Of course, such a tendency seems compatible with a solution-focussed approach in practise (e.g., call the chaplain).

It is important to note here, however, that this section does not contest solution-focused practise in EOL care, like Kollar's work (1997) on Solution Focused Pastoral Counselling (SFPC) and other short-term approaches when working with people towards the end of their life. This section simply identifies a controversy with which hospice practise presents itself, and draws on some thoughts about how this becomes challenging for service users, practitioners and the service all together.

Christian-centred lens

A different conclusion from this book is pertinent to Blumer's (1958) examination of race prejudice. Blumer (1958) asserted that prejudice is not inherent to the feelings of individuals, but is dependent on a group position. He suggests that 'one should keep clearly in mind that people necessarily come to identify themselves as belonging to a racial group; such identification is not spontaneous or inevitable but a result of experience' (Blumer, 1958, p. 3). Equally, if we explore this idea in relation to religion and faith more broadly, one's experience means that one identifies with a group, this identification being inherent to who one is, and therefore inevitably informing how one practises. In other words, unconscious bias and naturally practising through the lens of one group's understanding of faith when working with people from other faith backgrounds is not unexpected, however it is a challenge which hospice care has not yet resolved.

With this in mind, and treating hospice care as an organisation that identifies with Christianity because of experience (i.e., history and development) (see Chapter 1), the undeniable Christian-centred approach opens a whole discussion about whether professional practise is *neutral*, as suggested in death policies (see Chapter 3), or, at least at times, biased due to a Christian framework. Findings demonstrate that when the conversation is focussed on religion, hospice professionals in general (although there are exceptions) assume the discussion to be focussed on religions other than Christianity. This is strengthened by the biblical language that professionals use when informally and indirectly referring to service users – 'angels' in one example (also reported in Chapter 4).

This conclusion becomes more complicated when conceptualised through a religious literacy lens. Religious literacy, as it is addressed and applied in this book, seeks to equip professionals with the abilities and skills to engage with an increasingly diverse service user population. This is, nevertheless, accountable to the capacity of hospice professionals to consider themselves part of the diverse environment, rather than seeing themselves as the knowledgeable person, distant from the overall population, who will solve problems. As per Amiot and Bourhis' (2005) explorations of intergroup discrimination and the asymmetry effect, an attitude like the one described in this section poses dangers – predominantly, the risk of imposing discriminatory and prejudiced practise on service users. Elsewhere (Pentaris, 2018a), I have explored the impact of religious illiteracy in EOL care and concluded with three types of religious microinvalidations: verbal, non-verbal and environmental. Such microinvalidations inevitably influence the service user experience and affect quality of care.

Religious literacy model for hospice care

So far, this book has reported on empirical evidence which does not only show how current practise incorporates the religious, belief and spiritual identities of service users, but also highlights where the gaps are and how professionals could better prepare themselves to respond to such needs. Drawing on that knowledge, this section presents a religious literacy model for hospice care (RLHC). This model highlights in stages how hospice professionals can increase their religious literacy and, therefore, enhance the quality of services and the service user experience.

In Chapter 2, the diverse descriptors of religious literacy were examined: an increase in knowledge about religious traditions, knowledge about religions but lack of understanding of them, and a process through which professionals need to engage better with the information that makes them uncomfortable, to name a few. It is clear, not only from the variety of the ways in which religious literacy is understood, but also from the progression of this book's arguments, that religious literacy can only be understood in context. The context, inclusive of circumstances, content and intent, is imperative to comprehend how religious literacy fits into practise and for what reasons.

For the purposes of enhancing religious literacy in hospice care, the recognition of its relevance to the context and philosophy of hospices is of absolute importance. Equally, an understanding of the links between end of life and bereavement is critical; it will motivate organisations and professionals alike to enhance their skills and abilities in this area. The significance of developing religious literacy has been made clear elsewhere (Pentaris, 2018a). However, how are we to measure religious literacy to avoid constructively the impact of religious illiteracy?

The RLHC model's purpose is twofold: first, to offer practitioners, and hospice practise generally, a tool by which to measure necessary qualities when working with people for whom religion, belief and spirituality are important aspects. The second is to offer hospice care and policy-makers in EOL care a tool to set standards for practise. Also, the model helps distinguish between culture and religion, two concepts that may not be connected (Foucault, 2013 [1999]) but have often been used interchangeably.

Advancement of religious literacy

The advancement of religious literacy is a lifelong process, a journey which is never ending and in which professionals must constantly remain aware of their use of professional self when working with others. Specifically, this process is highly complicated and necessitates 'that professionals recognise a continuous need for ongoing understanding of religion and spirituality and are willing to involve their religious, nonreligious, or spiritual self in that process' (Pentaris, 2018b, n.p.).

The RLHC model consists of three stages, two of which are bound together: acquisition of knowledge about religion, belief and spirituality; understanding of one's knowledge and a phenomenological appreciation of the sense of meaning such identities offer; and, last, appropriate skills and abilities to engage with individuals for whom these identities are important. For this process to be successful, a value-based approach needs be employed and used as a lens through which hospice professionals can confidently approach the potential of increased religious literacy. Equally, from an organisational perspective, hospices can promote the advancement of religious literacy through such a lens. Figure 8.1 offers a brief visual of the model, whereas Figure 8.2 details the model and its stages.

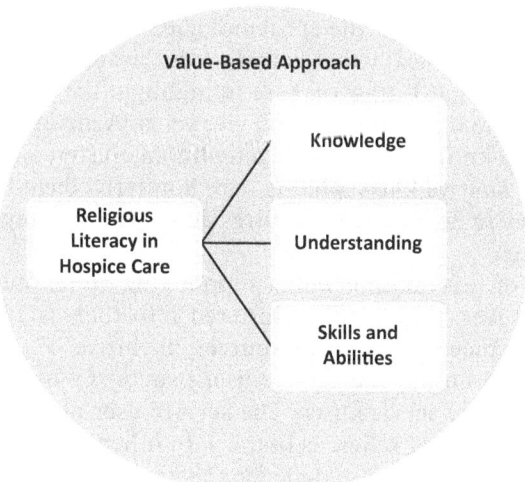

Figure 8.1 Religious literacy in hospice care

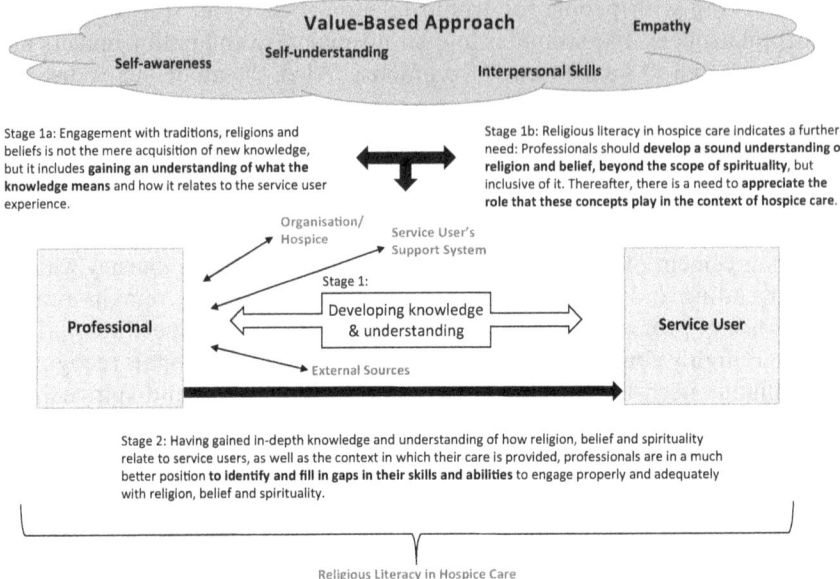

Figure 8.2 Model of religious literacy in hospice care

Knowledge

The procurement of new knowledge is not simply the process of receiving information, even though this is an important aspect of learning. New knowledge is also developed, and in various forms (Lehrer, 2018). In the sense of 'know' as *competence* and *information sharing*, as per Lehrer (2018), knowledge is also the product of interactions between people and their environment, between the epistemological (conceptual understandings) and the metaphysical (what is real). It is, however, the idea of skeptical epistemology that I draw on here to highlight the dubious nature of epistemology without metaphysics and vice versa. A metaphysical analysis would lead us to know what is real, yet with an epistemological analysis we can identify *how* we know what is real. Similarly, the advancement of religious literacy in hospice care requires developing a competence which benefits practise.

The sources of information which support the professional's learning vary a lot; however, they can be clustered into four categories: (1) the organisation/hospice; (2) external sources, inclusive of external training, books and so on; (3) the service user's support system (formal and informal) and (4) the service user. The service user plays a vital part in the process of advancing religious literacy. In other words, professionals' level of religious literacy is also dependent on how well they have engaged with the idea of learning from the service user. Equally, the development of further knowledge is dependent both on the professional's ability and willingness to receive new information from various sources, but also on the hospice organisation's willingness to offer the opportunities for professionals to do so.

Understanding

The enhancement of information, no matter how rich, becomes useless when there is no in-depth understanding of it – how and why it relates to the circumstances, the origins of the information and its influence on everyone involved. These are but a few of the questions which are pertinent to the process of increasing religious literacy.

Many philosophers and sociologists of knowledge and the science of knowledge (e.g., Kukla, 2013) have engaged in an inexhaustible dialogue about knowledge and its construction. Drawing on social constructivism (also see Kukla, 2013) and the idea of skeptical epistemology, the RLHC model upholds that the knowledge that professionals may receive from a service user, for example, must also be understood and put into context. To do so, professionals must develop a thorough understanding of the information, which is achieved through comprehending how a person's knowledge was constructed: social constructivism. In other words, receiving information about a religious tradition or a ritual – say, about what Buddhists do when someone dies or what Christians do when someone is grieving – is important, but incomplete in the process of advancing religious literacy. Professionals ought to examine the information from the service users' perspective and develop an understanding of what portion of the knowledge is relevant to them and what is not, how it relates to them and how it does not and so on. An equal process is necessary when working with individuals from a nonreligious, nonspiritual or nonfaith background.

Moreover, it is imperative that professionals grow their understanding of religion and belief beyond the scope of spirituality. The latter may be unlimited yet difficult to appreciate. Thereafter, there is a need to fathom the role these concepts play in the context of hospice care – from the inception of hospice care to its contemporary transformation.

Skills and abilities

Reminiscing Lehrer (2018), one way of understanding knowledge is to perceive it as *competence*:

> In one sense, 'to know' means to have some special form of competence. Thus, to know the guitar or to know the multiplication tables up to ten is to be competent to play the guitar or to recite the products of any two numbers not exceeding ten. If a person is said to know how to do something, it is this competence sense of 'know' that is usually involved. (Lehrer, 2018, p. 5)

Table 8.1 Quantifying religious literacy

Measures	Religious literacy	
	Description	Examples
Engagement with traditions, religions and beliefs	Engagement with traditions, religions and beliefs is not the mere acquisition of new knowledge. It includes gaining an understanding of what the knowledge means and how it relates to the service users' experiences.	Enlarge one's knowledge about various traditions to use as a canvas for further development. Employ a person-centred approach by which service users become the educators who inform the healthcare professional about the meaning their belief has to them and how it plays out with their experience. Conduct a spiritual needs assessment during admission that involves a discussion with the service user. Actively engage in conversations with service users to understand what their request (religious related) means to them. Set aside time to discuss service users' intervention plan through the lens of their belief system. Do not avoid questions or comments about religion and belief. Refer service users to the chaplain only upon request. Record spiritual needs and feed them to the multidisciplinary team (MDT) meeting.
Development of an understanding of religion and belief and their role in the context of hospice care	Religious literacy in hospice care indicates a further need: Professionals should develop a sound understanding of religion and belief beyond the scope of spirituality, but inclusive of it. Thereafter, there is a need for appreciating the roles these concepts play in the context of hospice care.	Familiarise oneself with hospice history and hospice ideology. Work with chaplains to gain further understanding of the role of faith in hospices. Participate in monthly focus groups to critically reflect on the roles of religion, belief and spirituality in hospice care, and exercise one's skills of talking about religion and belief.

Acquiring new knowledge, whether in a linear and non-interactive way, or through the process of connecting and interacting with others, suggests either the facility to develop a new skill or explore new abilities, or the development of a new skill itself.

This stage in the RLHC model does not suggest that skills and abilities develop naturally and without effort, simply as a consequence of receiving information. Lehrer (2018) asserted that knowing how to play the guitar, for example, indicates the competency to do so. However, one is as skilled to play the guitar as the hours spent practising. In other words, gaining new knowledge and developing an understanding of it can either become irrelevant because of the passing of time or be criticised as unnecessary, unless it benefits the skills and abilities of professionals in the field to work better with service users for whom religion, belief and spirituality are important. It is the ability to identify gaps in skills and competencies that is important in the first two stages of the model.

Table 8.1 offers some practical examples of how Stages 1a and 1b in Figure 8.2 can materialise.

Value-based approach

All the stages just discussed are best understood through the lens of a value-based approach that includes self-awareness, self-understanding, interpersonal skills, and empathy – all important aspects of professional development in hospice care (Table 8.2).

Table 8.2 Value-based approach

Value-based approach	
Measures	*Description*
Self-awareness	Professionals should develop the skill of introspection – the ability to recognise themselves as individuals separate from the wider context of the organisation.
Self-understanding	Self-understanding refers to the ability to reconceptualise oneself as part of a wider system and organisation. With self-awareness and self-understanding, professionals show understanding of their identities, as well as how they relate to the identities of other people.
Interpersonal skills	Interpersonal skills are essential when setting out to work with people. Excellent communications and listening skills best prepare professionals to respond to the religious (and nonreligious) diversified service user group in the hospice.
Empathy	The development of empathy and empathic approaches enhances the ability to build better and stronger rapport with people from different faiths and belief systems.

Concluding note

This chapter has done two things. First, it highlighted the key concepts that emerged from the previous sections in this book. Second, it presented a religious literacy model for use in hospice care. Discussion about both parts of the chapter does not come without challenges and perhaps limitations. I am not offering an exhaustive list of critiques here. Perhaps this is something for readers to do. I am, however, offering some reflections about how the RLHC model could play out in the community, especially considering the rise of compassionate communities as well as religious institutions in communities.

Sallnow, Bunnin and Richardson (2015) wrote:

> In the UK, the notions of hospice and community are closely intertwined at conceptual, strategic and operational levels. Many hospices in this country owe their origins, early funding and initial plans to local people or groups who had a vision to create a new service for people dying in their area and who were prepared to donate time, money and effort to make this vision a reality. Such community support remains vital for the majority of hospices even as they are well established and employ large numbers of professionals to deliver care and manage the business of the organisation. (Sallnow, Bunnin and Richardson, 2015, p. 1)

Despite the contrast between some of the ideas shared in this quote and some of this book's arguments, local communities have undeniably played an important role in the delivery of EOL care. More than 125,000 volunteers engage with hospice services in the community, for example (Help for Hospices, 2014).

Compassionate communities are found across Europe (also see Wegleitner, Heimerl and Kellehear, 2015) and their primary purpose is health promotion (Kellehear, 2013), even though responsibility for EOL care is now placed on everyone in the community, regardless of qualifications and expertise. This is, indeed, a deeply noble idea and perhaps carries with it principles from previous centuries. However, it also places more pressure on regulatory bodies of EOL care and hospice care specifically. If religious literacy is a pressing issue with hospice professionals who have at least basic education on professional – service user communication, compassion, empathy and person-centred care, it is imperative that religious literacy be introduced to all involved in the care of the dying and the bereaved.

Equally, religious literacy is neither palpable nor well-defined when it comes to religious institutions. Religious literacy, as discussed earlier in this book, is much more than knowing a lot about one or two religions. That said, religious institutions in the community, which contribute to compassionate communities and EOL care in the community more widely, may also be scrutinised for their level of religious literacy and potential for applying a model of religious literacy to increase understanding of faith and nonfaith, as well as develop further skills to engage efficiently with the diverse identities society presents itself with.

References

Amiot, C.E. and Bourhis, R.Y., 2005. Discrimination between dominant and subordinate groups: The positive–negative asymmetry effect and normative processes. *British Journal of Social Psychology*, 44(2), pp. 289–308.

Blumer, H., 1958. Race prejudice as a sense of group position. *Pacific Sociological Review*, 1(1), pp. 3–7.

Campbell, C.S., 2012. Boundary crossings: The ethical terrain of professional life in hospice care. In Smith, D.H. (ed.), *Caring well: Religion, narrative, and health care ethics*. Louisville, KY: Westminster John Knox Press, pp. 201–220.

Clines, J. with Gilliat-Ray, S., 2015. Religious literacy and chaplaincy. In Dinham, A. and Francis, M. (eds.), *Religious literacy in policy and practice*. Bristol, UK: Policy Press, pp. 237–256.

Cobb, M., Puchalski, C.M. and Rumbold, B. (eds.), 2012. *Oxford textbook of spirituality in healthcare*. Oxford, UK: Oxford University Press.

Day, A., 2011. *Believing in belonging: Belief and social identity in the modern world*. Oxford, UK: Oxford University Press.

Day, A., 2009. Believing in belonging: An ethnography of young people's constructions of belief. *Culture and Religion*, 10(3), pp. 263–278.

Department of Health, 2016. *Our commitment to your end of life care: The government response to the review of choice in end of life care*. London, UK: Department of Health.

Department of Health, 2008. *End of life care strategy: Promoting high quality care for all adults at the end of life*. London, UK: Department of Health.

Dinham, A. and Francis, M. (eds.), 2015. *Religious literacy in policy and practice*. Bristol, UK: Policy Press.

Dollard, J., 1983. *Toward spirituality: The inner journey*. Center City, MN: Hazelden Foundation.

Foucault, M., 2013 [1999]. *Religion and culture*. London, UK: Routledge.

Furness, S. and Gilligan, P., 2010. Social work, religion and belief: Developing a framework for practice. *British Journal of Social Work*, 40(7), pp. 2185–2202.

Gilliat-Ray, S., 2005. From "chapel" to "prayer room": The production, use, and politics of sacred space in public institutions. *Culture and Religion*, 6(2), pp. 287–308.

Help the Hospices, 2014. New exhibition showcases rich legacy of hospice volunteering. Press release, February. Available at: https://www.hospiceuk.org/media-centre/press-releases/details/2014/02/27/new-exhibition-showcases-rich-legacy-of-hospice-volunteering.

Hook, J.N., Davis, D.E., Owen, J., Worthington Jr, E.L. and Utsey, S.O., 2013. Cultural humility: Measuring openness to culturally diverse clients. *Journal of Counseling Psychology*, 60(3), pp. 353–366.

Hughes, M. and Wearing, M., 2017. *Organisations and management in social work*. Thousand Oaks, CA: Sage.

Kellehear, A., 2013. Compassionate communities: End-of-life care as everyone's responsibility. *QJM: An International Journal of Medicine*, 106(12), pp. 1071–1075.

Kollar, C.A., 1997. *Solution-focused pastoral counseling: An effective short-term approach for getting people back on track*. Grand Rapids, MI: Zondervan.

Kukla, A., 2013. *Social constructivism and the philosophy of science*. London, UK: Routledge.

Lehrer, K., 2018. *Theory of knowledge*. London, UK: Routledge.

Luker, K.A., Austin, L., Caress, A. and Hallett, C.E., 2000. The importance of 'knowing the patient': Community nurses' constructions of quality in providing palliative care. *Journal of Advanced Nursing*, 31(4), pp. 775–782.

McGuire, M.B., 2008. *Lived religion: Faith and practice in everyday life*. Oxford, UK: Oxford University Press.

McSherry, W., 2001. Spiritual crisis? Call a nurse. In Orchard, H. (ed.), *Spirituality in health care contexts*. London, UK: Jessica Kingsley, pp. 107–117.

Mladovsky, P., Rechel, B., Ingleby, D. and McKee, M., 2012. Responding to diversity: An exploratory study of migrant health policies in Europe. *Health Policy*, 105(1), pp. 1–9.

Nebel Pederson, S. and Emmers-Sommer, T.M., 2012. "I'm not trying to be cured, so there's not much he can do for me": Hospice patients' constructions of hospice's holistic care approach in a biomedical culture. *Death Studies*, 36(5), pp. 419–446.

Owens, A. and Randhawa, G., 2004. 'It's different from my culture; they're very different': Providing community-based, 'culturally competent' palliative care for South Asian people in the UK. *Health & Social Care in the Community*, 12(5), pp. 414–421.

Pentaris, P., 2018a. The marginalization of religion in end of life care: Signs of micro-aggression? *International Journal of Human Rights in Healthcare*, 11(2), pp. 116–128.

Pentaris, P., 2018b. Religion, belief and spirituality in healthcare. In Gehlert, S. and Browne, T. (eds.), *Handbook of Health Social Work (3rd edition)*. Somerset, NJ: John Wiley & Sons.

Pentaris, P., 2016. *Religious literacy in end of life care: Challenges and controversies*. Unpublished Doctoral Thesis (Goldsmiths, University of London).

Pentaris, P. and Thomsen, L.L., 2018. Cultural and religious diversity in hospice and palliative care: A qualitative cross-country comparative analysis of the challenges of healthcare professionals. *Omega: Journal of Death and Dying,* Accepted paper.

Sallnow, L., Bunnin, A. and Richardson, H., 2015. Community development and hospices: A national UK perspective. In Wegleitner, K., Heimerl, K. and Kellehear, A. (eds.), *Compassionate communities: Case studies from Britain and Europe*. London, UK: Routledge, pp. 1–14.

Watson, B., 2015. Can we move beyond the secular state? *Religions*, 6(4), pp. 1457–1470.

Wegleitner, K., Heimerl, K. and Kellehear, A. (eds.), 2015. *Compassionate communities: Case studies from Britain and Europe*. London, UK: Routledge.

Conclusions

Religion, belief, spirituality, faith or the lack of all the above – and many other ways in which people self-identify – are integral aspects of life. Such identities have, for centuries, offered the basis for shared values, norms, beliefs and collective mentalities which all lead not only to the formation but the advancement of societies. Sociology has best taught us this lesson (e.g., Scott, 2006), and if we pay close attention to the work of Auguste Compte's (Comte, 1855), one of the pronounced fathers of sociology from the 19th century, we will quickly realise that the focus on these characteristics is not only essential but inevitable. Expressly, Compte (1855) argued that humans differ from other animals on the basis of collective being, which is the product of linguistics. It is only with language, signs, symbols and the meaning attached to them that societies come together and are sustained. In other words, religion, belief and spirituality are a rich source of linguistics and meaning: associated factors in contemporary societies and individual consciousness.

Contemporary societies continue to grow in diversity and, consequently, complexity. To explain this better, different religions, spiritualities, secular identities and so on constitute a sense of collective being among the people who share such values, language and meaning. This is a 19th-century way of thinking, though. Currently, we are considering: How do people from different religions find peace in the same place, when the way they perceive, understand and experience the world is so different? This is a challenge that reflects Herbert Spencer's (1897 [1850]) ideal about industrial societies. From a state of aristocracy and hierarchy, we moved into a place where individuals acquired citizenship rights and gained power in their social roles. However, this book makes a slightly different argument – one which identifies a state of disequilibrium between the social classes in the cultural formation of hospice care.

To use a metaphor, drawing on Spencer's (1897 [1850]) suggestions, hospice professionals are the regulatory system, which acts as a reminder of the stratification of the dominant and subordinate groups in the care system, with the latter being service users and their families and friends. Not surprisingly in this metaphor, service users or families and friends are the subordinate groups which abide by the power structures developed and introduced by the regulatory system. Returning to the point about industrialisation, in this case, we are facing a paradox. Even though the subordinate system gained rights and a voice to express wishes and preferences, as well as have demands, the power structures which boost the imbalances we observe in Marxist societies remain. The combination of these two is incompatible, and this book concludes that the answer may be that we appreciated our skills and abilities to integrate with one another quite highly.

To position this conclusion better in the context of this book, it is important to return to our initial thesis. Given the shifting demographics of the population and, equally, the people who make use of services towards the end of their life, how do hospice professionals respond to the mix of religious, spiritual and nonreligious identities that have emerged in public in the past 20 years? Evidence shows that despite ongoing attempts to expand skills and knowledge in hospice care, services users or their allies often remain dissatisfied in the way their worldview is accommodated or treated. This book reached a conclusion that, in hospice care, we often manage needs following a more technical and business-oriented route. One thought that accompanies this conclusion is that, perhaps, we ought to consider further deconstructing what we know, or think we know, and learn anew. Perhaps the stories of the past cannot dictate the materiality of the future. I acknowledge the ambiguity in this thought. However, I invite readers to examine hospice care and the role and place of religion, belief and spirituality in it through the lens of Spencer's social evolution (Spencer, 1897 [1850]). This experience may help appreciate the need for more meaning-oriented rather than business-oriented practises.

Scott (2006) grasps Spencer's concept of evolution with accuracy:

> Spencer saw societies as systems that maintain an equilibrium state, much as organisms do. The actions of individuals as they pursue their goals move super-organic systems into equilibrium or disequilibrium with respect to their natural environment and the biological and psychological characteristics of their members. Disequilibrium consists of strains and tensions that pressurise individuals to act in ways that adapt their society to its environment and so re-establish equilibrium. The tendency to adaptation, therefore, is the means through which social systems change, and Spencer described this adaptive change as 'evolution'. (Scott, 2006, p. 31)

Drawing on this descriptor, this book concludes with the realisation that hospice care on the whole is still moving towards re-establishing equilibrium, from a religious and spiritual angle. There are additional actions required to perfect the balance between what we know and what is. To explain this further, I approach both aspects separately here.

First, in the previous chapter, I expanded on hospice professionals' willingness to engage well with religion and belief and commitment to quality care. However, willingness and commitment are both dependent on the way in which we comprehend them and equally appreciate the need to be willing and committed. Both concepts have, therefore, a reliant nature regarding professionals' education, training, background and expertise. The conclusions offered in Chapter 8 should be taken with caution, as the aim is not to criticise current practise and professional rigour, but to raise awareness of the incompatibility of current training, or lack thereof, in the areas of religion, belief and spirituality. The majority of professionals in hospice care are now individuals who were trained in the 1970s onwards. This coincides with the period when secularisation theories took hold, and the tendency to separate religion from public life was at the forefront of formulating practise. Especially younger professionals in hospice care may not have had the chance to train in this area properly, and this gap in educational programmes impacts on what they know.

Since the 2000s, the need to become more religiously and spiritually sensitive in practise became pertinent to professional life due to the shifting changes in the role of religion in society, as discussed in Chapter 2. In response to this need, hospice care embedded abundant study days to its culture and required professionals to approach this training with care. What becomes apparent now, though, is that the technical approach to training, which is reflected in Dinham and Francis' (2015) argument about the tendency to know more about more religions, offers a view of how different religious denominations approach death, dying and bereavement, but it neglects a central factor: lived belief.

Moving into the field now, it becomes clearer to many practitioners, researchers and policy-makers that religion, belief, faith and spirituality are lived experiences and, therefore, we are unable to generalise knowledge the way we thought or hoped we could. To conclude, what we know seems not to match what is needed by service users and family members or friends, and this is a state of disequilibrium.

The RLHC model aims at bridging this gap and offers a method by which hospice professionals may be able to come close to aligning their skills and abilities to what people – for whom religion, belief and spirituality are important aspects of their life – require of them. I am, however, as I have noted earlier in this book, mindful of the ambiguity of the concept of religious literacy and its ambitious character.

Dinham and Francis (2015, p. 270) conclude that religious literacy 'is best understood as a framework to be worked out in context. In this sense, it is better to talk of religious literacies in the plural than literacy in the singular'. The RLHC model then presents one religious literacy, one which responds to the foundational principles of hospice care, and EOL care altogether. With this in mind, this book is not in any way conclusive. It does, though, emphasise the need for further work in this area and extended exploration of how to parallel professional capacities and literacies with the shifting needs of the people who are using hospice services.

Reaching the end of this book, it is important to sustain a sense of practise- and policy-based implications. This will further help us appreciate not only some of the points made earlier in this section, but also the applicability of the RLHC model.

Implications for social policy

The links between social policy and professional practise are undeniably strong (Higham, 2006), whereas the process is, or at least should be, reciprocal – social policy informed by professional practise and vice versa. This book has unpacked a wide area of concern regarding the challenges that hospice professionals face in relation to religion, belief and spirituality. The findings are reflective and particularly tied to current death and health policies. It is also evident that technocratic theories (Hughes and Wearing, 2017) and materialised aspects of measurement for efficiency lead to misperceptions and misunderstandings, rather than sufficient and sensitive practise.

Dinham and Francis (2015, p. 257) conclude that religious literacy 'is a fluid notion'. Drawing from this, religious literacy in hospice care may only be conceptualised within the context in which it is perceived. In other words, the findings presented in this book may inform death and health policies in providing further insight to the implications of the mechanical language used to communicate service delivery on the front lines. This book can have a complementary role in all stages of social policy – planning, implementing, evaluating – with the following in mind. Hospice professionals consider policy documents detrimental to how, when and whether religion and belief have been integrated in EOL care. Furthermore, social policies add significance to the formation of ethical and timely professional practise. These two realisations are paramount to how the outcomes of this book can inform death and health policies.

An outstanding example of implication is the following. The *End of Life Care Strategy 2008* (Department of Health, 2008) is a document that requires revisiting and reconstructing of its content, despite the most recent advancements which complement the Strategy. Quality care, wellbeing, compassionate approaches, these are essential elements in the Strategy and the principles that truly guide the intentions of EOL care. The findings presented here can inform areas of the Strategy that apply either directly to how hospice professionals respond to religion, belief and spiritual identities of service users, or indirectly but efficiently to all areas in relation to quality care and enhancing the service user experience.

It is worth recognising here, however, the risk of conflict between religious literacy's fluidity and social policy's need for transparency and precision. Iatridis (2005), among other scholars, suggests that social policy documents need to be clear, as well as accurate. Policy sources that fail to address an issue directly and provide explicit guidelines about how to meet people's needs (also see Alcock, 2014), also fail to be applied successfully.

In consideration of this, the need to operationalise religious literacy is apparent. The main characteristics that have been identified in this book, and which shape religious literacy as a more measurable and tangible outcome, are the following: engagement with traditions, religions and beliefs; and developing understanding of religion and belief and their role in the context of hospice care. As explored in Chapter 8 with the RLHC model, both features are best understood and applied through the lens of a value-based approach.

It is important to understand that despite the religious reference of the concept of religious literacy, its operationalisation is not centred on religion. As Pentaris (2016) has shown, professionals appear to demonstrate limited skills of interpersonal care when they mostly feel uncomfortable or in a situation in which they lack knowledge or understanding. A policy which addresses this is also a policy that comprehends the value of professionals' self-awareness and self-understanding. Responding to a service user group from a multi-faith environment is essentially associated with demonstrating the right skills to respond, appropriately, to diversity – an area that social policy has, so far, done well in, but with room for improvement. Equality Act 2010, for example, is inclusive of all public bodies and promotes equality whilst it recognises human rights. Nevertheless, the Act's aim remains exclusive of reducing inequalities, which inevitably lead to experiences of social exclusion in hospice care (e.g., Cohen, 2008).

Planning social policy is a process that requires multiple resources (Iatridis, 2005). An ever-changing society is one of the primary resources in this case. Ongoing adaptation to the new changes that are faced in EOL care are also indicators for social policy planning. This book reports on findings that present current self-understanding and professionalism in EOL care. These conclusions are part of the changes that shall become informers of new and restructured social policies in the area.

Implications for professional practise

Professional practitioners handle continuous education and adapt to a life-long learning approach to better equip themselves according to the ongoing changes in society. Religion and belief have seen tremendous change over the past few decades, as was explored in Chapter 2, and this change is subject to consideration when it comes to efficient, adequate and quality practise.

Health and social care literature (Hall and Roussel, 2012; Melnyk and Fineout-Overholt, 2011; McSherry, 2001) is representative of the significance of evidence-based practise. Professional practise ought to be informed by evidence and vice versa. It is real-time experiences that can better inform practise that successfully meets the needs of service users – similar to what Crisp (2008) suggests about subjective experience and its significance in a lifelong learning attitude. It is also worth adding that evidence is strained by time and space, which reinforces the need for lifelong learning approaches.

Religious literacy may be used as a framework to engage better with the new and challenging faith needs of service users, as well as to understand spiritual care better. In other words, compartmentalise and reconstruct it as part of care that hospice professionals can more comfortably understand and assimilate. It is the acquisition of the right language that is important in order to be able to engage with such needs. Evidently, this is a task that directly links to the education of professionals. Religious literacy may be an effective framework in which practise can further develop. However, the educational system shall be following same tactics for the hospice professionals to experience consistency and cohesiveness throughout their lifelong learning, including education and practise.

Final thoughts

Religion and belief are undeniably important aspects of people's lives, whether religious, nonreligious or secular. As such, they play a critical part in the way people appreciate their dying and grief, the way they approach the end of their life. That said, carers – both professional and non-professional – ought to take religion, belief and spirituality into account when providing their services. To do so, it is reasonable to turn our attention to the service users and start learning from them what their faith and belief mean to them and how they shape their experiences. This requires an open mind, lack of humility and a commitment to lifelong learning.

References

Alcock, P., 2014. *Social policy in Britain*. Hampshire, UK: Palgrave Macmillan.

Cohen, L.L., 2008. Racial/ethnic disparities in hospice care: A systematic review. *Journal of Palliative Medicine*, 11(5), pp. 763–768.

Compte, A., 1855. *The positive philosophy of Auguste Comte*. New York, NY: Calvin Blanchard.

Crisp, B.R., 2008. Social work and spirituality in a secular society. *Journal of Social Work*, 8(4), pp. 363–375.

Department of Health, 2008. *End of life care strategy: Promoting high quality care for all adults at the end of life*. London, UK: Department of Health.

Dinham, A. and Francis, M. (eds.), 2015. *Religious literacy in policy and practice*, Bristol, UK: Policy Press.

Hall, H.R. and Roussel, L., 2012. *Evidence-based practice: An integrative approach to research, administration, and practice*. Burlington, MA: Jones & Bartlett.

Higham, P., 2006. *Social work: Introducing professional practice*. Thousand Oaks, CA: Sage.

Hughes, M. and Wearing, M., 2017. *Organisations and management in social work*. Thousand Oaks, CA: Sage.

Iatridis, D.S., 2005. *Οργανισμοί κοινωνικής φροντίδας [Social care organisations]*. Athens, Greece: Ellinika Grammata.

McSherry, W., 2001. Spiritual crisis? Call a nurse. In Orchard, H. (ed.), *Spirituality in health care contexts*. London, UK: Jessica Kingsley, pp. 107–117.

Melnyk, B.M. and Fineout-Overholt, E. (eds.), 2011. *Evidence-based practice in nursing & healthcare: A guide to best practice*. Baltimore, MD: Lippincott Williams & Wilkins.

Scott, J., 2006. *Social theory: Central issues in sociology*. Thousand Oaks, CA: Sage.

Spencer, H., 1897 [1850]. *Social statics*. New York, NY: Appleton.

Index